D0894363

WESTERN IOWA TECH

Uniformed Services Nursing

Guest Editors

DEBORAH J. KENNY, PhD, RN,
Lieutenant Colonel, US Army (retired)
BONNIE M. JENNINGS, DNSc, RN, FAAN,
Colonel, US Army (retired)

NURSING CLINICS OF NORTH AMERICA

www.nursing.theclinics.com

Consulting Editor
SUZANNE S. PREVOST, RN, PhD, COI

June 2010 • Volume 45 • Number 2

6-10-10   Ebsco BPo#8035 $45⁵⁰

SAUNDERS an imprint of ELSEVIER, Inc.

WESTERN IOWA TECH-LIBRARY

W.B. SAUNDERS COMPANY

A Division of Elsevier Inc.

1600 John F. Kennedy Blvd., Suite 1800 • Philadelphia, PA 19103-2899

http://www.theclinics.com

NURSING CLINICS OF NORTH AMERICA Volume 45, Number 2
June 2010 ISSN 0029-6465, ISBN-13: 978-1-4377-1841-6

Editor: Katie Hartner
Developmental Editor: Donald Mumford

© **2010 Elsevier Inc. All rights reserved.**

This journal and the individual contributions contained in it are protected under copyright by Elsevier, and the following terms and conditions apply to their use:

Photocopying
Single photocopies of single articles may be made for personal use as allowed by national copyright laws. Permission of the Publisher and payment of a fee is required for all other photocopying, including multiple or systematic copying, copying for advertising or promotional purposes, resale, and all forms of document delivery. Special rates are available for educational institutions that wish to make photocopies for non-profit educational classroom use. For information on how to seek permission visit www.elsevier.com/permissions or call: (+44) 1865 843830 (UK)/ (+1) 215 239 3804 (USA).

Derivative Works
Subscribers may reproduce tables of contents or prepare lists of articles including abstracts for internal circulation within their institutions. Permission of the Publisher is required for resale or distribution outside the institution. Permission of the Publisher is required for all other derivative works, including compilations and translations (please consult www.elsevier.com/permissions).

Electronic Storage or Usage
Permission of the Publisher is required to store or use electronically any material contained in this journal, including any article or part of an article (please consult www.elsevier.com/permissions). Except as outlined above, no part of this publication may be reproduced, stored in a retrieval system or transmitted in any form or by any means, electronic, mechanical, photocopying, recording or otherwise, without prior written permission of the Publisher.

Notice
No responsibility is assumed by the Publisher for any injury and/or damage to persons or property as a matter of products liability, negligence or otherwise, or from any use or operation of any methods, products, instructions or ideas contained in the material herein. Because of rapid advances in the medical sciences, in particular, independent verification of diagnoses and drug dosages should be made.

Although all advertising material is expected to conform to ethical (medical) standards, inclusion in this publication does not constitute a guarantee or endorsement of the quality or value of such product or of the claims made of it by its manufacturer.

Nursing Clinics of North America (ISSN 0029-6465) is published quarterly by Elsevier Inc., 360 Park Avenue South, New York, NY 10010-1710. Months of issue are March, June, September, and December. Periodicals postage paid at New York, NY and additional mailing offices. Subscription price per year is, $133.00 (US individuals), $306.00 (US institutions), $228.00 (international individuals), $374.00 (international institutions), $184.00 (Canadian individuals), $374.00 (Canadian institutions), $70.00 (US students), and $115.00 (international students). To receive student/resident rate, orders must be accompanied by name of affiliated institution, date of term, and the signature of program/residency coordinator on institution letterhead. Orders will be billed at individual rate until proof of status is received. Foreign air speed delivery is included in all *Clinics* subscription prices. All prices are subject to change without notice. **POSTMASTER:** Send address changes to *Nursing Clinics*, Elsevier Health Sciences Division, Subscription Customer Service, 3251 Riverport Lane, Maryland Heights, MO 63043. **Customer Service: Telephone: 1-800-654-2452** (U.S. and Canada); **1-314-447-8871 (outside U.S. and Canada). Fax: 1-314-447-8029. E-mail: journalscustomerservice-usa@elsevier.com** (for print support) and **journalsonlinesupport-usa@elsevier.com** (for online support).

Nursing Clinics of North America is covered in *EMBASE/Excerpta Medica, MEDLINE/PubMed (Index Medicus), Social Sciences Citation Index, Current Contents, ASCA, Cumulative Index to Nursing, RNdex Top 100,* and Allied Health Literature and International Nursing Index (INI).

Printed in the United States of America.

WESTERN IOWA TECH-LIBRARY

Contributors

CONSULTING EDITOR

SUZANNE S. PREVOST, PhD, RN, COI
Associate Dean, Practice and Community Engagement, University of Kentucky,
Lexington, Kentucky

GUEST EDITORS

DEBORAH J. KENNY, PhD, RN, LIEUTENANT COLONEL, US ARMY (RETIRED)
Beth El College of Nursing and Health Sciences, Colorado Springs, Colorado

BONNIE MOWINSKI JENNINGS, DNSc, RN, FAAN, COLONEL, US ARMY (RETIRED)
Evans, Georgia

AUTHORS

ANDRES AZUERO, PhD
Assistant Professor, Department of Nursing, University of Alabama, Birmingham, Alabama

CAPT ANA MARIE BALINGIT-WINES, MPA, RN, USPHS, CC
Senior Regulatory Officer, Office of Compliance, Center for Devices and Radiological
Health, Food and Drug Administration, Silver Spring, Maryland

CDR MICHELLE BRAUN, MSN, CRNP, USPHS, CC
Nurse Practitioner, Kidney Disease Section, National Institutes of Health, Clinical Center,
Bethesda, Maryland

LTCOL MICHAEL BROTHERS, PhD, USAF
Director, USAF Academy Human Performance Laboratory, United States Air Force
Academy, Colorado

TSUI-LAN CHOU, MSN, RN
Supervisor, Nursing Department, SongShan Armed Forces General Hospital, SongShan
District, Taipei City, Taiwan, Republic of China

MARY PAT COUIG, MPH, RN, FAAN, REAR ADMIRAL, USPHS (RETIRED)
Bethesda, Maryland

CDR DAVID R. CRUMBLEY, MSN, RN, NC, USN
National Naval Medical Center, Bethesda, Maryland

CAPT ANNETTE TYREE DEBISETTE, PhD, RN, USPHS, CC
Senior Regulatory and Science Training Officer, Food and Drug Administration, Office
of Regulatory Affairs, Division of Human Resource Development, Rockville, Maryland

CAPT THOMAS L. DOSS, RN, MPH, USPHS, CC
Utilization Review/Quality Assurance Nurse, TRICARE Management Activity, Office of the Assistant Secretary of Defense (Health Affairs), US Department of Defense, Falls Church, Virginia

PAO-LUO FAN, MMM, MD
Director Lieutenant General, Medical Affairs Bureau, Ministry of National Defense, Taipei, Taiwan, Republic of China

LTC DAWN M. GARCIA, RN, MHA, CCRN, FACHE, AN, USA
Head Nurse, Critical Intensive Care Unit, Landstuhl Regional Medical Center, Landstuhl, Germany

COL KATHRYN M. GAYLORD, PhD, RN, AN, USA
Research Investigator, Director of Provider Resiliency Program, United States Army Institute of Surgical Research, Fort Sam Houston, Texas

CURTIS HOBBS, MD, COLONEL, US ARMY (RETIRED)
Endocrinologist, Department of Medicine, Madigan Army Medical Center, Tacoma, Washington

LI-YUAN HO, MSN, RN
Director, Nursing Department, SongShan Armed Forces General Hospital, Songshan District, Taipei City, Taiwan, Republic of China

CDR MICHELE A. KANE, PhD, RN, NC, USN
National Naval Medical Center, Bethesda, Maryland

CHI-WEN KAO, PhD, RN
Assistant Professor, School of Nursing, National Defense Medical Center, Taipei, Taiwan, Republic of China

MAJ ANN KOBIELA KETZ, MN, AN, USA
Clinical Nurse Specialist, Medical Surgical Unit, Landstuhl Regional Medical Center, Landstuhl, Germany

RDML ANN R. KNEBEL, DNSc, RN, FAAN, USPHS, CC
Deputy Director for Preparedness Planning, Office of the Assistant Secretary for Preparedness and Response, US Department of Health and Human Services, Washington, DC

CAPT CAROL L. KONCHAN, MSN, CRNP, USPHS, CC
Nurse Practitioner, National Institute of Neurological Disorders and Stroke, National Institutes of Health, Bethesda, Maryland

CAPT ANGELA LACEK, RN, BSN, MSHS, USAF, NC
Clinical Nurse, Family Medicine, 87th Medical Group, McGuire Air Force Base, New Jersey

DI LAMB, BSc (Hons), MA, PMRAFNS, SQUADRON LEADER, RAF
Aeromedical Evacuation Cell–OC PA/AELO, The Royal Centre for Defence Medicine, Selly Oak Hospital, Birmingham, United Kingdom

LORI A. LOAN, PhD, RNC
Chief, Nursing Research Service, Madigan Army Medical Center, Tacoma, Washington

LTC LEONARDO M. MARTINEZ, MPH, RN, AN, USA
Chief, Preventive Medicine, DeWitt Health Care Network, Fort Belvoir, Virginia

KATHLEEN D. MARTIN, MSN, RN, CCRN
Trauma Program Nurse Director, Joint Theater Trauma System, Landstuhl Regional Medical Center, Landstuhl, Germany

CAPT ANGELA M. MARTINELLI, PhD, RN, CNOR, USPHS, CC
Health Science Administrator, Division of Treatment and Recovery Research, National Institute on Alcohol Abuse and Alcoholism, National Institutes of Health, Rockville, Maryland

MARY S. MCCARTHY, PhD, RN, CNSN, MAJOR, US ARMY (RETIRED)
Clinical Nurse Researcher, Nursing Research Service, Madigan Army Medical Center, Tacoma, Steilacoom, Washington

CAPT SUSAN ORSEGA, MSN, CRNP, USPHS, CC
Nurse Practitioner, Division of Clinical Research, Collaborative Clinical Research Branch, National Institute of Allergy and Infectious Disease, National Institutes of Health, Bethesda, Maryland

LTCOL KATRINA POOLE, RNC, BSN, MA, USAF, NC
Flight Commander, Perinatal Unit, Elmendorf Air Force Base Hospital, Elmendorf Air Force Base, Alaska

MARY CANDICE ROSS, PhD, RN, COLONEL, US AIR FORCE (RETIRED)
Professor and Associate Dean for Faculty Development, College of Nursing, Florida State University, Tallahassee, Florida

LTC MARIA SERIO-MELVIN, MSN, RN, CCRN, AN, USA
Clinical Nurse Specialist, United States Army Institute of Surgical Research, Fort Sam Houston, Texas

LTC NANCY M. STEELE, PhD, RNC, WHNP, AN, USA
Chief, Europe Regional Medical Command, Nursing Research, Landstuhl Regional Medical Center, Landstuhl, Germany

COL ELIZABETH A.P. VANE, MSN, RN, AN, USA
Assistant Professor, Perioperative Clinical Nurse Specialist Program, Graduate School of Nursing, Uniformed Services University of the Health Sciences, Bethesda, Maryland

KWUA-YUN WANG, PhD, RN
Deputy Director, Nursing Department, Taipei Veterans General Hospital; Professor, School of Nursing, National Defense Medical Center, Taipei, Taiwan, Republic of China

MAJ CANDY WILSON, PhD, ARNP, USAF, NC
Director of Nursing Research, Wilford Hall Medical Center, Lackland Air Force Base, San Antonio, Texas

COL THOMAS G. WINTHROP, MSN, RN, AN, USA
Chief of Perioperative Services, Walter Reed Army Medical Center, Washington, DC

MAJ SHANNON WOMBLE, MSN, CCNS, ACNP, USAF, NC
Assistant Head Nurse and Critical Care Clinical Nurses Specialist, Critical Intensive Care Unit, Landstuhl Regional Medical Center, Landstuhl, Germany

MAJ HAZEL WRIGHT, MSN, MSED, ARNP, RN-BC, USAF, NC
Chief, Staff Development, Education Division, Landstuhl Regional Medical Center, Landstuhl, Germany

MEEI-HORNG YANG, MSN, RN
Director, Nursing Department, Wei-Gong Memorial Hospital, Taiwan, Republic of China

LINDA H. YODER, PhD, MBA, RN, AOCN, FAAN, COLONEL, US ARMY (RETIRED)
Luci Baines Johnson Fellow in Nursing, Associate Professor, University of Texas at Austin School of Nursing, Austin, Texas

Contents

> Iron deficiency is recognized as a significant health concern for women of childbearing age in the civilian population. In the military, most women are of childbearing age. Not only do they carry the normal risks for developing iron deficiency, but they also have the added threats of possible decreased choices of food high in iron content, increased physical activity, and weight loss. This can put these women at risk for decreased energy efficiency and impaired cognitive performance. This article describes the pathophysiology of iron deficiency and iron deficiency anemia, the consequences of each, and the need to routinely screen military women for iron depletion.

> This article highlights the potential negative effect of the current combat environment on bone health of young military men and women who may be at risk for stress fractures and future bone disease because of alterations primarily in diet and physical activity level during deployment. A combination of physiologic biomarkers, including bone turnover and bone mineral density, and nutrition and exercise surveys can provide meaningful data on potential health risks related to deployment. Soldiers participating in an investigation into bone health before and after deployment did not have decreased bone density but the study did raise awareness about an issue that might otherwise go unnoticed because preventive care is typically focused on older adults. Several risk factors may be modifiable and nurses have the necessary skills for counseling and monitoring behaviors that can minimize disabling musculoskeletal injuries that affect quality of life for the individual and unit readiness for the commander.

> The US Public Health Service (PHS) is one of 7 uniformed services operating for the nation. Nurses form the largest category of personnel in the PHS and are integral members of teams identified to deploy in times of national need. PHS nurses serve "in harm's way" to protect and defend the public

health of the nation during national emergencies and disasters of great magnitude, such as 9/11, Hurricane Katrina, the H1N1 virus outbreak, and so forth. In this article, the authors discuss how active-duty Commissioned Corps nurses in the US PHS respond during times of national need. Military nurses may be asked to serve in war zones, participate in humanitarian missions, and care for military beneficiaries. By contrast, the role of nurses in the Commissioned Corps is to protect, defend, and advance the public health of the nation. PHS nurses are critical members of interdisciplinary health care teams organized to provide health care to diverse populations in the United States and abroad.

The events of September 11, 2001, set in motion the broadest emergency response ever conducted by the US Department of Health and Human Services. In this article, some of the nurses who deployed to New York City in the aftermath of that horrific attack on the United States offer their recollections of the events. Although Public Health Service Commissioned Corps (PHS CC) officers participated in deployments before 9/11, this particular deployment accelerated the transformation of the PHS CC, because people came to realize the tremendous potential of a uniformed service of 6,000 health care professionals. When not responding to emergencies, PHS CC nurses daily serve the mission of the PHS to protect, promote, and advance the health and safety of the nation. In times of crisis, the PHS CC nurses stand ready to deploy in support of those in need of medical assistance.

Since the beginning of the wars in Iraq and Afghanistan, the incidence of pressure ulcers from various causes has increased. This article discusses the knowledge nurses need to care for casualties returning from Operation Iraqi Freedom (OIF) and Operation Enduring Freedom (OEF) who may be at risk for developing pressure ulcers. This article also describes the development of an evidence-based pressure ulcer awareness program for young adults aged 18 to 35 years at a military treatment facility that receives casualties from OIF/OEF. This evidence-based program enables nurses to rapidly assess casualties for risk factors and initiate nursing interventions to mitigate the development of pressure ulcers. Improving the detection of pressure ulcers among the young OIF and OEF casualties may, in turn, reduce mortality and morbidity among these service members.

Competencies for military nurses are much broader in scope than their civilian counterparts. Not only must they be proficient at basic nursing skills, but they must also quickly master such military skills as protecting themselves and others during attack or threat of attack, caring for major trauma victims under austere conditions, and preparing such patients for transport through the military system of evacuation. This requires consistent and specialized training. This article describes the competencies necessary for practice by military nurses.

Severe Acute Respiratory Syndrome (SARS) had an enormous effect on Taiwan's public health and the nation's economy. To prevent the spread of the epidemic, the government implemented strategies and measures for the control of the epidemic. The Ministry of National Defense also fully supported epidemic prevention by mobilizing all necessary human and material resources. Under the plan executed by the Ministry of National Defense, the SongShan Armed Forces Hospital became Taiwan's first hospital dedicated exclusively for the treatment of patients with SARS. Uniformed Service Nurses' devoted to caring for patients with SARS during the outbreak made significant contributions to the prevention and control of SARS.

This article describes the experiences of two obstetric nurses as they deployed to the war zone in Iraq. Each discusses her role as a medical-surgical nurse and an emergency room nurse, respectively, and how she dealt with learning to practice in these areas. Each nurse came away from the experience with newfound confidence in her abilities and an appreciation for flexibility in practice. They also describe the challenges of deployment and being away from family, and how they coped with their feelings associated with nursing in a war zone and caring for injured service members and the indigenous population.

Since the beginning of the Overseas Contingency Operation, more than 45,000 ill and wounded service members have been evacuated from the battlefield to Landstuhl Regional Medical Center (LRMC) in western Europe. LRMC is a stopover for these service members, where they are further assessed, treated, and stabilized before they return to the United States. This process requires coordination between different military services, health care teams, and modes of transportation. These processes can be complicated given the severity of the wounded. Nurses at LRMC have learned how to streamline services, providing efficient, comprehensive care for wounded service members and their families.

Infections, troublesome in even optimal health care environments, can be a source of serious and persistent concern for local populations and health care workers during a disaster, and in austere environments such as those found in Iraq and Afghanistan. For these scenarios, it is vital to have standard infection control practices in place and to have them used consistently. Only then will healthcare workers be able to contain the potential spread of disease and improve conditions for those affected.

Nursing plays a critical role in the comprehensive burn care delivered at the US Army Institute of Surgical Research, otherwise known as the US Army's Burn Center serving the Department of Defense. This center serves as a model for burn units nationally and internationally. It also provides a challenging and innovative work environment for military and civilian nurses. Nurses in the Burn Center contribute to innovations in acute, rehabilitative, and psychological care for patients with burns. This article provides an overview of the complex nursing care provided to burn patients treated at the Burn Center.

Modern warfare has generated a significant increase in blast injuries, which demand careful management during planning and while undertaking air transfer. Pain management following multiple injuries can be challenging even when a patient is cared for in a stationary health care setting; this is further complicated by the additional stressors of flight. This article describes health care governance initiatives implemented by the Aeromedical Evacuation Squadron, based at Royal Air Force (RAF), United Kingdom. It focuses on quality and performance improvements via a program of clinical-effectiveness auditing.

THE CLINICS ARE NOW AVAILABLE ONLINE!

Access your subscription at:
www.theclinics.com

Preface

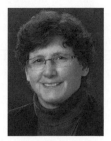 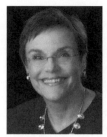

Deborah J. Kenny, PhD, RN,   Bonnie M. Jennings, DNSc, RN, FAAN,
Lieutenant Colonel, US Army (retired)   Colonel, US Army (retired)
Guest Editors

There are 3 military services in the United States—the Army, the Navy, and the Air Force. Nurses who join the military wear the uniform of their respective service. Nurses may also join the United States Public Health Service (USPHS). They wear the uniforms of the USPHS and, as such, they are a part of the uniformed services although they are not part of the military.

Although nurses in the uniformed services have responsibilities similar to nurses who work in civilian settings, nurses in uniform also have unique roles in caring for unique patient populations in distinctive care environments. The patients are typically people who need health care because they have experienced extreme conditions. The conditions could be the result of natural disasters, such as earthquakes, hurricanes, or tsunamis, in which case the nurses are a part of a humanitarian mission. The conditions could be the result of decisions to engage in conflicts throughout the world, as in Iraq or Afghanistan, in which case nurses are working in a war zone or a combat setting. The care environments can range from facilities that look and function like civilian hospitals to tents or even open-air setups. Equipment can range from state-of-the art, highly effective field equipment to older or even more makeshift paraphernalia. Either way, training is required for nurses to learn how to use the equipment.

At the outset of humanitarian or combat missions, nurses find themselves working in a primitive environment. Nurses have described trying to care for patients in blowing sand, in extreme heat and cold, and while protecting themselves and their patients as they heard rocket fire overhead. As time goes on, the environment "matures" and becomes less austere, better organized, and better equipped. Despite the range of environments and maturation, uniformed nurses have a remarkable sense of duty when asked to perform whatever roles they are assigned; these roles are sometimes different from those in which they have specialized. This issue of *Nursing Clinics of North America* illustrates some of the roles that uniformed nurses fulfill and their dedication to those for whom they care.

Although joined by the bond of serving their country, each of the US uniformed services has its own culture, which includes a language that may be difficult to understand by those not familiar with it. This is more than a uniformed/civilian dichotomy. These are cultural and language issues that make it difficult for the various uniformed

Nurs Clin N Am 45 (2010) xiii–xv
doi:10.1016/j.cnur.2010.03.011
0029-6465/10/$ – see front matter © 2010 Elsevier Inc. All rights reserved.

nursing.theclinics.com

services to understand one another's policies, language, and acronyms. For instance, those serving in the Army are called soldiers; Air Force personnel are referred to as airmen; and those in the Navy are sailors. Collectively, military personnel are called service members. Each service also has its own names and abbreviations for different ranks.

There are 2 large clusters of military personnel: officers and enlisted. Individuals who have a minimum of a baccalaureate degree may choose to become commissioned as officers. As they progress in rank, officers are given increasing leadership roles, beginning with small groups and often culminating in positions in which they are in charge of thousands of service members. Nurses are officers. Individuals who join the military after high school enlist; these individuals are referred to as "enlisted" personnel while they are in the most junior ranks. Once enlisted personnel are promoted to a certain rank, regardless of service affiliation, they become known as noncommissioned officers (NCOs). The NCOs have more responsibility and are often in charge of a group of enlisted service members. They also assist the officers and are regarded as the backbone of military units. Some NCOs continue their education and have various college degrees. Unless they choose to embark on the process to become an officer, however, they remain NCOs. The USPHS comprises entirely commissioned officers and they provide a distinctive service for the United States. Their missions are usually more related to humanitarian efforts and maintaining security within the United States rather than serving in combat zones.

Distinctions among the military services continue into the combat environment, also called the theater of operations. Ill or injured members from any service, however, including the Marine Corps, may be treated at a facility or by the staff from any service. Army hospitals are called Combat Support Hospitals (CSH); the acronym is pronounced, "cash." Military health care personnel in a CSH treat service members with minor wounds and return them to duty; they stabilize service members with serious injuries or illness for evacuation out of theater. Air Force mobile hospitals are called field hospitals. Although the Air Force has hospitals on the ground in combat zones, their primary mission in a war zone is to evacuate patients to Europe or the United States for definitive care and rehabilitation. Critically injured patients are escorted from the theater of operations by a critical care air transport team (CCATT), called a C-Cat. Most CCATT members are Air Force, although infrequently some team members may be Army. The Navy also has units on the ground, called military hospitals. The primary Navy operations take place on ships, such as the US Navy Ship (USNS) Comfort or the USNS Mercy. These ships are located near the theater of operations. In Iraq and Afghanistan, as well as the major military hospital in Europe, it is common to see a mixture of Army, Navy, and Air Force personnel working side by side, in one hospital, regardless of its name, mixing their different cultures. Everyone shares the goal of providing the best care possible for ill and injured service members.

This issue of *Nursing Clinics of North America* is dedicated to the nurses in the uniformed services. It highlights some of the unique roles uniformed nurses play that put them in unique circumstances. Within this issue, the nurse authors of some articles discuss personal accounts of the situations they were in as a result of their uniformed responsibilities. Knebel and colleagues speak to the role of USPHS nurses in the rescue and recovery operations after the 9/11 attack on the World Trade Center. The authors reveal many of the sensory phenomena they encountered. Poole and Lacek discuss how, as nurses who specialized in obstetrics and gynecology, they quickly accommodated to very different roles when they deployed to Iraq. They portray how they coped with learning to care for severely injured patients and the pride they felt in their accomplishments.

Because uniformed nurses often deploy to assume responsibilities other than those in their area of expertise, 2 articles in this issue address competencies needed to perform these unique duties. Ross describes competencies and skills needed for nurses who deploy. Debisette and colleagues offer examples of some of the missions and roles with which the nurses in the USPHS are involved.

Other articles in this issue discuss common conditions that have unique implications for uniformed nurses. For instance, Wilson and Brothers address iron deficiency anemia; McCarthy and colleagues describe calcium losses. These common conditions take on a unique set of considerations when viewed from a military perspective. Likewise, Crumbley and Kane discuss the relatively common occurrence of pressure ulcers. They do so, however, from the perspective of young, healthy men and women who have been injured and develop pressure ulcers due to the injury or ischemia associated with blood loss or because of the field conditions during the initial insult. Vane and colleagues put a new perspective on the common problem of infection control by commenting on ways to minimize the transmission of infection in austere field conditions.

In another group of articles, the authors describe systems that augment care for military members injured in combat zones. Steele and colleagues describe the care provided for service members as they make their way from the battlefields, through Germany, to definitive care in the United States. Serio-Melvin and colleagues discuss care for severely burned service members, with attention to ways continuity is ensured across the care continuum.

Although most of the articles written for this issue are by uniformed nurses from the United States, 2 articles were included to offer a voice from military nurses abroad. Chou and colleagues discuss what military nurses in Taiwan endured, physically and psychologically, during the 2004 severe acute respiratory syndrome epidemic. Lamb describes how nurses managed the pain experienced by injured British soldiers as they were air evacuated by the Royal Air Force from the theater of operations.

This broad range of articles offers a good look at what nurses in uniform are called to do and under what conditions they must practice. Readily apparent in each of these articles is the intense loyalty these nurses felt toward their patients and their mission. Like those who served before them, these nurses are continuing the legacy of uniformed nurses called to work in war zones and disaster areas. They do so proudly and with courage. We are honored to present their work to you.

ACKNOWLEDGMENTS

The above Guest Editors would like to acknowledge the TriService Nursing Research Program (TSNRP) for its assistance in the preparation of this issue of *Nursing Clinics of North America*.

Deborah J. Kenny, PhD, RN, Lieutenant Colonel, US Army (retired)
Beth El College of Nursing and Health Sciences
1420 Austin Bluffs Parkway
Colorado Springs, CO 80918, USA

Bonnie M. Jennings, DNSc, RN, FAAN, Colonel, US Army (retired)
4211 Sutter's Court
Evans, GA 30809, USA

E-mail addresses:
dkenny@uccs.edu (D.J. Kenny)
bmjennings@knology.net (B.M. Jennings)

Erratum

Refers to:
Preface
By Karren Kowalski
March 2010 Volume 45 Issue 1
ISSN 0029-6465

In the March 2010 issue of *Nursing Clinics of North America*, an error was made in the Preface. That article should have been credited to both Guest Editors of that issue: Patricia S. Yoder-Wise and Karren Kowalski.
   We apologize for this oversight.

Nurs Clin N Am 45 (2010) xvii
doi:10.1016/j.cnur.2010.01.001
0029-6465/10/$ – see front matter © 2010 Elsevier Inc. All rights reserved.

nursing.theclinics.com

Iron Deficiency in Women and Its Potential Impact on Military Effectiveness

Candy Wilson, PhD, ARNP[a],*, Michael Brothers, PhD[b]

KEYWORDS

- Military • Iron deficiency • Women's health • Iron screening
- Risk factors • Iron deficiency anemia

In 1993, the Presidential Commission on the Assignment of Women in the Armed Forces rescinded the risk rule, which had prohibited women in the US military from serving in certain positions based on a substantial risk of capture.[1] Lifting this ban allows today's military women to serve in positions that historically had not been open to them, such as aviator, navigator, mechanical technician, infantry, gun crew, just to name a few of the historically all-male military positions.[2] Today, more women are choosing to join the military and are serving their nation with a greater choice of military occupations.

Women make up 14% of the US military population, with the US Air Force having the highest proportion of women: 19%.[3] In Iraq and Afghanistan combined, 10% of those serving in the military are women.[4] The increased number of women has required the military medical system to assess the health care services provided in both the continental United States and in rugged settings abroad, whether in deployed or humanitarian settings. These services must be delivered in the context of differences by gender in health and illness so as to maintain a fit and ready force. Fortunately, research that examines and sheds insight into the salient differences in health care needs between men and women is burgeoning. Some health care conditions, such as iron deficiency (ID), are more prevalent among women than among men. ID can reduce the oxygen-carrying capacity of blood, in turn impairing optimal physical and cognitive functioning. The high prevalence of ID in military women parallels the high prevalence of this problem in women athletes, and this must be

[a] Nursing Research, Wilford Hall Medical Center, 2200 Bergquest Drive, Building 4430, Lackland Air Force Base, TX 78236-9908, USA
[b] United States Air Force Academy Human Performance Laboratory, 2169 Field House Drive/Suite 111, United States Air Force Academy, CO 80840, USA
* Corresponding author.
E-mail address: Candy.wilson@lackland.af.mil

Nurs Clin N Am 45 (2010) 95–108
doi:10.1016/j.cnur.2010.02.005
0029-6465/10/$ – see front matter. Published by Elsevier Inc.

considered a condition that warrants regular screening to help ensure the optimal performance of military women. ID is defined by the Centers for Disease Control and Prevention (CDC) as "an abnormal value for at least two of the following three indicators: serum ferritin, transferrin saturation, [or] free erythrocyte protoporphyrin."[5] Those with ID who also have a low hemoglobin value (<12 g/dL) are considered to have ID anemia (IDA).[5]

It is widely known that women are diagnosed with IDA at a far higher rate than are men,[6] and ID continues to be identified as a health concern primarily for women. For those in the military, having ID can be detrimental to completing their mission because of its potential to restrict physical and cognitive functioning.[6,7] However, the true prevalence of ID in women serving in support of Operation Iraqi Freedom/Operation Enduring Freedom (OIF/OEF) has not been published.[8]

Women who voluntarily join the US Armed Forces (Army, Navy, Air Force, Marines) represent all racial, ethnic, and socioeconomic backgrounds, and more than half are aged 18 to 24 years.[9] Unfortunately, women of childbearing age, a category that includes the great majority of military women, are at the greatest risk for ID.[6] This is important, because undiagnosed and untreated ID can become IDA, which could affect the military mission negatively by making women unable to perform at optimal levels.

To date, the iron status of military women has not been explored systematically on a population basis. Few data exist to determine the relationship between blood mineral levels and performance in military women, but this relationship has been studied in similar nonmilitary populations.[8] The purposes of this article are to present relevant research and clinical knowledge regarding the sequelae of ID, to propose that additional clinical resources be allocated to routinely screen for this condition, and to ask for continued research on the effectiveness of screening and clinical interventions, especially during physically strenuous missions.

THE DEFINING CHARACTERISTICS OF ID

Patients with ID can vary from being completely asymptomatic to having symptoms similar to anemia, such as weakness, headache, irritability, varying degrees of fatigue, and exercise intolerance.[10] Women who undergo intense military physical and mental training, however, are likely to dismiss these vague symptoms as a result of exhaustion from their training. A physical assessment for people with chronic ID can include evaluating the patient for the symptoms described above and for glossitis, angular stomatitis, koilonychia (spoon nails), blue sclera, esophageal webbing (Plummer-Vinson syndrome), and anemia. Abnormal food cravings, known as pica, also can be exhibited by people with ID, who may resort to eating dirt (geophagia) and ice (pagophagia) without an apparent biologic reason for these cravings.[11]

THE PHYSIOLOGY OF IRON ABSORPTION

In people, iron is obtained in two ways: absorption from foods in the gastrointestinal (GI) tract and recovery from senescent and damaged erythrocytes.[12] Iron obtained from the GI tract is absorbed in the first section of the duodenum, a highly acidic environment that is necessary for the membrane iron transporters.[12] There are two types of dietary iron: heme and nonheme. Heme iron already has been incorporated into the heme molecules—hemoglobin and myoglobin—both of which are absorbed well in the body. Most of the Western population's consumption of iron in food is nonheme iron found in plant foods and fortified food products. Indeed, only about 10% of the iron in the typical Western diet is heme iron, which is derived from meat, poultry, and fish.[13]

The bioavailability of nonheme iron is variable and depends on the current diet and the amount of iron already present in the body.

Regardless of the type of iron consumed, the minimum daily dietary requirement for this mineral among women aged 19 to 30 years is 18 mg/d.[5] Nonheme iron is less readily absorbed, and its absorption is strongly influenced by the other foods ingested at the same meal.[6] Foods or beverages high in bran, dietary fiber, calcium, tannins (in tea and coffee), oxalates, phylates, and polyphenols (in certain plant-based foods) can interfere with absorption. Foods rich in ascorbic acid (vitamin C), such as citrus fruit, broccoli, mango, pineapple, and guava, in contrast, will facilitate the absorption of iron.[6] Additionally, foods rich in heme iron promote the absorption of nonheme iron.

Iron that is not needed immediately is stored in ferritin molecules, primarily in the liver, bone marrow, and spleen.[13] A single ferritin molecule holds up to 4500 atoms of iron.[12] In a healthy person, most of the iron in the body is conserved and reused. Although iron losses are usually minimal, they do occur through the GI tract, skin, urine, and with menstruation.[13]

PATHOPHYSIOLOGY OF ID

In people, a decline in iron status occurs in stages and is usually gradual. If not treated, it can progress from iron depletion, to iron-deficient erythropoiesis, and finally to IDA.[6] The decline develops when the iron demand is not met by available iron, resulting in insufficient iron for the synthesis of hemoglobin.[14] The iron and hemoglobin deficiency eventually will produce iron-deficient red blood cells.[10]

A normal laboratory serum ferritin level ranges from 40 to 160 µg/L for females; iron depletion is reflected by a serum ferritin between 12 and 20 µg/L. In ID, the serum ferritin is less than 10 µg/L up to 12 µg/L, a level at which the stores are considered to be exhausted.[13,15] ID is diagnosed when the depletion of iron stores begins to impair the synthesis of hemoglobin.[13] If the negative iron balance is not corrected, the final stage of ID is IDA, which is known as one of the microcytic anemias, in which the red blood cells look pale and small.[13]

DIAGNOSTIC EVALUATION

Asking people to recall their diet is not an effective method of screening for ID and cannot substitute for further testing, if warranted.[13] The gold standard for identifying ID or IDA is a direct test bone marrow biopsy with Prussian blue staining, but this test is not practical for screening.[13] The complete blood count (which includes the hematocrit, hemoglobin concentration, mean corpuscle volume, and red blood cell distribution width) is the basic measurement for determining the late stages of ID or IDA.[13] Serum biochemical markers, as will be described, such as serum ferritin, serum iron, total iron-binding capacity, transferrin saturation, serum transferrin receptor, and zinc protoporphyrin/heme, are helpful in identifying ID before the onset of IDA. Normal and abnormal values are depicted in **Table 1**. Serum biochemical markers include:

> Serum ferritin is an early marker of ID and is highly specific for this condition. Serum ferritin is the storage compound for iron, and low levels correlate with a diagnosis of ID.[16] However, other conditions can alter the serum ferritin levels, such as inflammation, chronic infection, and other diseases.
> Serum iron concentration, which can be measured directly, generally decreases as iron stores are depleted. The ideal serum iron concentration is greater than 115 µg/dL. The serum iron concentration also can be influenced by extraneous factors such as iron absorption from meals, infection, inflammation, and diurnal variation.

Laboratory Test	Normal Range	Iron Deficiency	Iron Deficiency Anemia
Hematocrit	38–50%	38–50%	<38%
Hemoglobin	12–16 g/dL	12–16 g/dL	<12 g/dL
Red blood cell volume distribution width (RDW)	≤15%	>15%	>15%
Mean corpuscular volume (MCV)	80–100 fL	Normal range or <80 fL	<80 fL
Total iron binding capacity (TIBC)	330 ± 30 mcg/dL	360–410 mcg/dL	≥410 mcg/dL
Ferritin	100 ± 60 ng/mL	≤20 ng/mL	<12 ng/mL
Iron	115 ± 50 µg/dL	<115 µg/dL	<40 µg/dL
Soluble transferrin receptor	<35 mg/dL	≥35 mg/dL	≥35 mg/dL
Transferrin saturation	35 ± 15%	<20%	<10%
Zinc protoporphyrin/Heme	<40 µmol/mol	≥40 µmol/mol	≥70 µmol/mol

Table 1
Laboratory analysis for identifying iron deficiency and iron deficiency anemia

Total iron-binding capacity (TIBC) measures the availability of iron-binding sites. Extracellular iron is transported in the body bound to transferrin, a specific carrier protein. Therefore, TIBC indirectly measures transferrin levels, which increase as the serum iron concentration decreases. This test has lower values in the presence of conditions such as malnutrition, inflammation, chronic infection, and cancer.

Transferrin saturation (Tfsat), which indicates the proportion of occupied iron-binding sites, reflects iron transport rather than storage. Tfsat is calculated by dividing the serum iron concentration by TIBC. A low Tfsat implies low levels of serum iron relative to the number of available iron-binding sites, which suggests low iron stores. Tfsat decreases during the iron-deficient stage and is less sensitive to changes in iron stores than serum ferritin.

Serum transferrin receptor (TfR) is present on the reticulocyte membrane. With iron deficiency in the tissues, there is a proportional increase in the number of transferrin receptors. TfR is useful as an early marker of ID, and it is also helpful in differentiating between IDA and anemia of chronic disease (this test is not readily available in the military health care system).

Zinc protoporphyrin (ZPP) is formed when zinc is incorporated into protoporphyrin in place of iron during the final step of heme biosynthesis. Normally, the reaction with iron predominates, but when iron is in short supply, the production of ZPP increases, and the ZPP/heme ratio (reported as ZPP) becomes elevated. ZPP is elevated in the setting of lead poisoning and chronic disease. A newer hematologic test, reticulocyte hemoglobin content, may help diagnose ID before anemia is present.[13]

PREVALENCE OF ID

ID is a common diagnosis worldwide.[16] Interestingly, it is the only nutrient deficiency of significant prevalence in the developed nations.[6] In the United States, the Healthy People 2010 report called for a reduction in ID in children and pregnant women. In order to collect data for the prevalence of ID in the US population, the CDC uses the National Health and Nutrition Examination Survey (NHANES), which relies on a nationally representative sample of the US civilian noninstitutionalized population.[17] In the third NHANES (NHANES III, 1988 to 1994), researchers found that 11% of female adolescents (ages 16 to 19 years) but less than 1% of male adolescents had diagnostic symptoms of ID.[18] In addition, 3% of female adolescents had diagnostic symptoms of IDA. The next age group of women, ages 20 to 49, had an incidence of ID equal to that of the adolescent girls, 11%, but their incidence of IDA was 5%. Among military women, one study found a 13.4% prevalence of ID at initial entry into military service, but following military basic training for 9 weeks, the prevalence increased to 32.8%.[19] Women in the US military who are aged 18 to 24 years are at equal or greater risk for developing ID/IDA based on the risk factors summarized in the next section.[9]

RISK FACTORS FOR ID IN WOMEN

Women at the greatest risk for ID are those who suffer with a chronic illness, experience heavy menstrual blood loss (>80 mL/month), or who are underweight or malnourished. This at-risk population should be screened.[10] Additionally, donating blood puts women at risk for ID.[15] Because requirements for military recruitment and retention limit and often restrict military service for women with chronic disorders, chronic illness and digestive illness will not be discussed as a cause of ID in this article. Also, for this article, it is assumed that military women are typically at their adult height, and thus growth spurts will not be covered as a contributor to ID in this population. In brief, the topics covered in this section will be limited to factors that render the military women in general at risk for ID.

Loss of Blood Through Menstruation

Women of childbearing age are at increased risk of ID because of monthly blood loss from menstruation. In a cross-sectional study of 335 premenopausal women in New Zealand, researchers found that women with a longer duration of menstrual flow (5.2 days) were more likely to be diagnostic of ID than were women with a shorter duration (4.9 days).[15] Proportionately, more women with a shorter duration of menstruation took oral contraceptives than the group with longer duration. In this study, diagnosis of ID was more common among women who did not use oral contraceptives (72.4%).

Experts recommend that oral contraceptives be used to treat ID,[20] but there are several other hormonal contraceptives that are an ideal reversible contraceptive method to decrease menstrual blood loss, particularly for women who wish to preserve their fertility. In addition to all combined oral contraceptive pills, examples include the levonorgestrel intrauterine system (Mirena; Bayer Health Care Pharmaceuticals, Wayne, NJ, USA), the etonogestrel contraceptive implant (Implanon; Schering-Plough Corporation, Kenilworth, NJ, USA), and injection with medroxyprogesterone acetate (Depo Provera; Pfizer, New York, NY, USA). With the exception of certain oral contraceptives, all the methods listed here are available to military women on request.

Race/Ethnicity

Researchers reporting results from NHANES III (1988 to 1994) and NHANES for 1999 to 2000 found that the prevalence of ID in these two studies was greater in non-Hispanic African American (15% to 19%) and Mexican American (19% to 22%) females than in non-Hispanic white (8% to 10%) females.[5] IDA is also more prevalent among women of color. For example, in a national survey, researchers reported much higher IDA rates for non-Hispanic African American (12.2%) and Mexican American (7.6%) females than for non-Hispanic white (2.6%) females.[21]

In a study of 1216 US Army women, differences in ID between racial/ethnic groups were consistent with other national studies. In this study, upon entry into military service, African American women were more likely to be diagnosed with ID (16.7%) than were white (8.9%) or Hispanic (7.1%) women.[19] At the conclusion of 9 weeks of physically and mentally intense basic military training, however, the rates of ID among all three racial/ethnic groups had increased. The greatest increase in prevalence was in the Hispanic women (a rise of 43.8%), followed by African American (up 32.5%), and white (up 24.8%) women.[19] Even though all women are offered the same meals in the military cafeterias during training, this does not mean that consumption is equal. The lack of cultural or personal food choice preferences in the cafeteria setting may be a possible contributor to women choosing not to eat the food that is offered.

Weight

In a New Zealand study of 335 women, researchers found that women with a body mass index (BMI, the weight in kilograms divided by height in meters squared) of less than 20 were more than twice as likely to be diagnosed with ID as women with normal BMI.[15] In a US study, the prevalence of ID among new military recruits who were underweight (BMI $\leq$19) was 18.3%.[22] Women should be encouraged to maintain a healthy weight and consume calories according to their activity level.

Military members of both genders serving in deployed locations are at risk for substantial and unintentional weight loss due to the lack of access to their personal food preferences, increased physical and emotional stress, and increased demands on their physical energy. Anecdotally, members of the military have verified weight loss associated with a recent deployment; this weight loss can come with a price of insufficiencies in micronutrients.[8] In addition, experts reported that under field conditions, with either field rations or with fresh foods, military members' serum ferritin decreased.[23] It is unclear why ferritin levels would decrease in the field environment, but this finding suggests an elevated incidence of ID, although to the authors' knowledge, ID has never been measured or reported among military members in this environment.

Dietary Choices

For whatever reason, many women do not consume the recommended daily reference intakes (DRI) of 18 mg/d of iron as established by the Food and Nutrition Board of the Institute of Medicine (National Academy of Sciences).[24] Also at risk for ID are those women who make restrictive diet choices, such as vegetarians.[10] There are no statistics on the number of military women who eliminate certain foods from their diets, but given the worldwide mobility of today's military, women who are deployed may be offered limited food choices based on what is immediately available.

Variety in food intake usually depends on how long military personnel are in a deployed location and the resources available for food preparation. The serving of food can vary from a buffet-style cafeteria with many options to a "meal ready to eat" (MRE) consisting of dried and canned foods in a pouch preserved for long shelf life and devoid of many natural nutrients found in fresh food. The usual food choice in the early stages of a humanitarian or contingency operation is MREs. The contents of these meal pouches are based on the dietary needs of the average male military member, however. Each MRE contains 7 to 9 mg of iron and will average around 1300 calories. Women in equal field conditions with similar activity levels do not need as high a caloric intake as men, and many will limit the number of meals they consume and, therefore, reduce their intake of iron below the DRI.

In 2006, the Institute of Medicine committee[8] reported a paucity of appropriately designed studies to give an accurate estimation of needs for iron in deployed locations, but it surmised that during deployment military members are highly active and experience increased iron loss through sweat and thus need more dietary intake of iron.[8] It is the recommendation of the Institute of Medicine[8] that women in military training or who are deployed receive 24 mg/d of iron due to the increased losses.[8] Interestingly, the Nutritional Standards for Operational Rations set the minimum daily requirement lower at 15 mg/d, 3 mg below the DRI.[8]

Donation of Blood

At times, members of the military may be called upon to donate blood for banking, or sometimes they simply take it upon themselves to give blood. After the national attack on Sept. 11, 2001, hospital employees and military members stationed at military treatment centers set up donation centers, and military personnel came in large groups to donate blood without prompting. This description of blood donation in times of crisis is not isolated to certain military bases, as such selfless acts have taken place across many military installations worldwide. Such altruism, however, can place women who may already have ID at further risk. Prior to donation, the blood banks check the hematocrit of their potential donors, and if is above 36% the candidate is approved for donation. The hematocrit, however, is a poor marker of hematological health overall. Moreover, in the New Zealand study, women who donated blood within the previous 4 months were seven times as likely to have decreased iron stores as women who had not donated, and they were more likely to be diagnosed with ID.[15] With this reported increased risk of ID following blood donation, it is interesting to note that in its 2006 report, "Mineral Requirements of Military Personnel," the Institute of Medicine did not describe the effects of blood donation on military personnel and did not recommend tighter surveillance of military members who donate blood.[8] Regardless, because of the substantial likelihood of developing ID from recent blood donation, military medical treatment facilities should screen for ID in women who have recently donated, and these women should be monitored by military medical professionals.

Physical Training

Because of the physical fitness requirements for the military, an overview of the risk factors for ID in athletes is relevant to this discussion. These risk factors include poor iron intake and restrictions on diet, increased erythropoiesis/turnover of red blood cells, GI blood loss, iron losses in sweat, foot-strike hemolysis, and thermohemolysis.[25,26] Athletes participating in impact sports have a greater prevalence of ID than those in nonimpact sports.[27,28] In one study, researchers reported that 36% of aerobically fit females had ID as compared with only 6% of their male counterparts.[29] Runners appear to have the highest incidence of ID, which is due to hemolysis from striking the foot.[26] Physical fitness assessments in the military rely heavily on the member's running time, but anaerobic measurements are taken also.

In a small study of Israeli female military recruits (average age 18 years), researchers reported an alarming rate of iron depletion (the serum ferritin level was <20 µg/L for 77% of women tested).[30] Furthermore, 10% of those women were found to have ID (ferritin level <12 µg/L). Elsewhere, in a double-blind, placebo-controlled study under way at the US Air Force Academy (USAFA) in Colorado Springs, Colo., researchers found that 14% of the female freshman cadets arrived at USAFA with a serum ferritin level below 12 mg/dL, while nearly 43% additional freshman women had a value below 20 mg/dL, suggesting that over half of these female recruits entered the military with either outright ID or in an iron status that placed them at risk for ID.[31] These female volunteers were randomly assigned to cohorts receiving either a daily pill containing 100 mg ferrous sulfate or a daily placebo, with instructions to take one pill every day. Following 6 weeks of basic military training at moderate altitude (the USAFA is approximately 7000 feet above sea level), over 55% of the subjects receiving the placebo had a serum ferritin value below 20 mg/dL, and nearly half had ID or IDA. None of the subjects receiving the daily iron supplement had IDA, however, although three could still be classified as iron depleted based on serum ferritin values above 12 but below 20 mg/dL. Although both groups displayed significant gains in total hemo-globin mass and blood volume, which would be expected when training at altitude, no significant differences in blood measures were evident within the first 10 weeks at alti-tude between the iron and placebo cohorts.[31] Statistically significant differences in blood volume and total hemoglobin mass became apparent as the year progressed, however, with the placebo group having lower blood values and worse exercise performance. Additionally, female subjects not receiving iron supplementation required a significantly longer time to fully adapt to USAFA's altitude, based on numerous measured blood parameters that included total hemoglobin mass, which was measured using the optimized CO (carbon monoxide) rebreathing protocol.[31]

In another study, this one of women in the US Army, researchers found that the prev-alence of ID had jumped from 13.4% at the beginning of training to 32.8% at the end.[19] They attributed this dramatic increase to physical activity and a possible decrease in dietary iron. Earlier, Beard and Tobin observed that the prevalence of ID was likely to be higher in athletic women than in sedentary women.[11] The causes for the increased prevalence are speculative but are likely related to dietary choices and to increased turn-over rates of both red cell and whole-body iron.[11] These speculations on the increased prevalence of ID among athletic women can be applied to military women in training because of the intense physical exercise necessary at that stage of military service.

EFFECTS OF ID ON PHYSICAL PERFORMANCE

As noted earlier, physical training can cause military women to develop ID, but the effects of ID on fitness also must be considered. Those who have ID can experience a substantial reduction in their capacity to exercise, a fact that creates a vicious cycle until the person is treated and the negative iron status is eliminated. ID alters exercise performance because of the decrease in oxygen transport to exercising muscle.[11]

Women working in certain military positions are required to perform at a physical fitness level that is comparable to that of men because of the demands of the position. Some military positions require fitness standards that are "normed" to the job (in these cases, men and women are expected to perform equally), such as a US Air Force aviator.[32] ID interferes with women's ability to perform at that capacity. In the Institute of Medicine's 2006 report "Mineral Requirements of Military Personnel," researchers reported that having IDA limits physical endurance.[8] The reduced levels of serum iron and the lower capacity of iron-dependent muscles contribute to lower endurance and energy inefficiency.[8] The recommendation by the Institute of Medicine regarding the impact of ID on performance was that military personnel be screened for iron status.[8]

EFFECTS OF ID ON EMOTIONAL/COGNITIVE PERFORMANCE

The connection between ID and impaired emotional status and reduced cognitive performance is convincing and deserves further investigation. In an Iranian study, researchers reported that female medical students diagnosed with depression had a mean serum ferritin level of 27.0 plus or minus 11.3 μg/L, well below the mean value of those who were not depressed: 38.4 plus or minus 17.1 µg/L ($p<.05$). The women in this study with ID were diagnosed with depression at a rate twice that of women without ID.[33] This connection between ID and depression is concerning and is relevant for military personnel. More recently, researchers reported that mental disorders were more common among women (9.0%) than men (5.7%) in Operation Iraqi Freedom.[34] Finally, McClung and colleagues[35] reported recently that iron supplementation for women with ID improved their mood and physical performance during military training in comparison with a group receiving placebo.

Reduced intellectual performance is a well-known and serious consequence of prolonged ID in children.[6] This consequence indicates that we should be concerned about young women with prolonged ID. Experts have reported overwhelming evidence that iron supplements given to women with ID improved both their learning and memory.[13,14]

THE EFFECT OF ID ON ADJUSTMENT TO ALTITUDE

People who travel to high altitudes (>9000 feet above sea level) generally experience weakness and anorexia during their initial adjustment to the altitude as well as other problems.[36] Weight loss is common with chronic exposure to high altitude until people become adjusted, and this loss of weight may be associated with an inadequate diet of iron-rich foods. In a retrospective study of male and female USAFA cadets, Brothers and colleagues[37] found that cadets who came to this moderate-altitude military academy from a location that was less than 900 feet above sea level demonstrated significantly lower aerobic and anaerobic physical fitness scores for 2 years when they were compared with those who came from locations with a moderate altitude (4500 to 9000 feet). This prolonged adjustment to altitude, when coupled with the presence of ID, is a concern because of ID's known effect on endurance capacity and energy levels.[8] In addition, Brothers and colleagues found that roughly one third of cadets coming from sea level (both male and female) experienced a drop in serum ferritin values to below 20 mg/dL. This drop in serum ferritin suggested that iron intake, although exceeding the DRI values, was insufficient for the erythropoietic demands of acclimatization to altitude. Physiologic adjustment to acclimatization, which produces a ferritin deficit, combined with the demanding military training environment, may have been a key reason for the protracted period of acclimatization and poorer athletic performance for up to 2 years. In the deployed setting, this combination of acclimatization to altitude and the presence of ID can be a hazardous combination, putting the health of the women and their military mission at risk.

A follow-up prospective study that included both male and female cadets (although only the data for males have been published thus far) from either sea level or moderate altitude produced the same results as summarized here, with former sea-level residents displaying significantly worse exercise performance for their first year at altitude.[38,39]

ID AND HEMORRHAGE

In any military conflict or training exercise, there is a risk of serious harm from hemorrhagic injuries. Clearly, women in such a setting who suffer from depleted or deficient iron stores are at a disadvantage compared with those who are not iron deficient. Although conceptually one can understand the risk of decreased oxygen-carrying capacity to vital organs that results from ID combined with hemorrhagic injury, a MedLine keyword search by the authors using the search terms of "iron deficiency," "iron deficiency anemia," "injury," and "hemorrhage" found no cross-matched articles from the year 1950 to the present that were relevant to the topic of hemorrhage in the setting of ID. However, researchers conducting a retrospective study on occult bleeding following trauma found that lower hemoglobin levels ($\leq$10 g/dL) in the early stages of hemorrhage were associated with an increased heart rate, decreased blood pressure, decreased pH, worsened base deficit, and increased requirements for transfusion.[40] Therefore, one could logically argue that the physiologic effects of hemorrhage might be exacerbated by the presence of ID. Certainly, decreased organ perfusion coupled with lower oxygen-carrying capacity could have serious consequences.

RECOMMENDATIONS FOR SCREENING

Whether screening for ID is cost-effective is a controversial issue among health care experts. Currently, there is no recommendation to screen for ID in women who are involved in intense military training or deployment. In addition, in a review of the literature, experts reported there was no compelling evidence from a preventive point of view to screen for iron in athletes.[41] Although recent research demonstrated an unexplained decline in the prevalence of IDA among US women, the prevalence of ID was unchanged; women with ID would still be at risk for worsening of that condition and possible IDA if the ID was uncorrected.[21] Researchers from two different studies attributed ID in female athletes and female military recruits to menstruation, inadequate dietary iron intake, GI bleeding, foot-strike hemolysis, sweat losses, and malabsorption of iron.[30,42] According to the US Preventive Services Task Force, there is at least fair evidence to support the screening of pregnant women for IDA to improve their health outcomes.[43] There is, however, no national standard to screen women for ID per se, and, therefore, there is not enough evidence to support the need for population screening. Experts in athletics, however, recommend the screening of elite athletes. In summary, the evidence presented here clearly indicates the need to screen for ID among military women, especially those who are in demanding physical situations or who are deployed for long periods of time or to higher altitudes.

NURSING CONSIDERATIONS

Nursing interventions for ID should be focused on educating the patient about the need to eat iron-rich foods. In addition, education should inform women about the signs and symptoms of ID. Nursing interventions also should include education on improving the uptake of iron while minimizing its loss. The fact that foods high in vitamin C interact with foods containing moderate-to-high levels of iron to increase uptake of the iron should be addressed.[15] Another key intervention is discussing options for minimizing menstrual blood loss among women for whom this is a problem.[15] Although information on suppressing menstruation is focused on the benefits of not having to manage menstruation while deployed, nurses should include the improvement of iron status as a second benefit of menstrual suppression.[20] It should be noted that despite the proactive campaign to educate military women about the beneficial effects of suppressing menstruation through hormonal contraceptives, military women continue to report their concern about the safety of this practice.[44] Nurses should reinforce the fact that menstrual suppression is a safe practice in order to dispel any myths or misconceptions.

Iron supplements provide the greatest improvement in iron status for women aged 19 to 50 years, of whom a reported 23% prophylactically supplement with iron. Groups at the greatest risk for ID (ie, low-income and minority women), however, are often least likely to consume iron supplements, and the dose of iron in multivitamins that contain this element is not sufficient for iron replacement in women with

ID.[16,45] Women who are prescribed iron supplements, typically an iron salt such as ferrous sulfate, should be warned of the typical GI side effects (such as constipation, dark or green stools, diarrhea, nausea, upset stomach, vomiting, and flatulence) to promote compliance with this therapy.[16] Teaching women about keeping their stools soft by using stool softeners and increasing fiber and water is an important intervention. Nurses need to ensure that follow-up testing of iron status is done every 3 to 6 months while women are on iron supplements.

Nursing considerations include educating health care colleagues about the generalized and vague symptoms that can be reported by athletic, military women that can be mistaken for the effects of intense physical training. This concern is especially important if there is a history of ID or, more importantly, IDA. Nurses should advocate for women who consistently score poorly on the physical fitness tests and consider screening them for the symptoms of ID and testing their iron status.

RESEARCH NEEDS

Given the high number of women who are diagnosed with conditions that could be the result of ID, additional research is needed in situations that simulate the deployed environment. Although population statistics are available along with a limited number of studies from military samples to demonstrate the prevalence of ID in women, the authors believe ID is underdiagnosed. ID is most likely dismissed because the usual tests by health care providers for its symptoms, such as fatigue, will not typically include a panel of the tests for iron listed previously. The amount of time needed to obtain results for an iron study panel can vary from laboratory to laboratory, but it is often quite substantial. Thus, the research community should be challenged to develop rapid and cost-effective screening methods for meeting the needs of the female military population.

Additional intervention studies are needed to test the appropriate intervention methods for women with ID in the deployed setting. Although the Institute of Medicine speculated in 2006 about the correct DRI for physically active women, there are unique risk factors for military women in a deployed setting that can place these women at greater risk for ID.[8] Therefore, research studies are needed to find the appropriate iron intake for women who are deployed. Some studies have examined iron supplements, and others have looked at improved iron intake through the diet. However, both interventional methods must be tailored to the deployed setting, which can vary in terms of the availability of supplements and foods.

Although the Institute of Medicine committee reported a decreased need for iron requirements for women on oral contraceptives, the committee did not outline the iron needs of women on a regimen of menstrual suppression.[8] This information would be helpful to inform women about the benefits of menstrual suppression that exist in addition to the obvious benefits of no menses and the decreased symptoms related to premenstrual changes.

SUMMARY

With the military population consisting of more women than ever before in US history, it is incumbent on military and health care leaders to explore the effect of ID on women, who are more at risk than men. Although the prevalence of ID in the deployed setting has not been published, based on populations similar to military women in training as well as studies of such women (female military trainees) one can speculate that the prevalence of ID in the deployed setting is between 11% and 43.8%. This high prevalence can be detrimental to the military mission, as the usual symptoms of ID are weakness, headache, irritability, fatigue, and exercise intolerance. The symptoms of ID can be exacerbated at deployed locations with moderate or high altitudes, such as northern Iraq and Afghanistan. Furthermore, the degree to which ID might exaggerate injury from hemorrhagic trauma is unknown, but it is speculated that women with ID who suffer such trauma might take longer to reach a stable state. Nursing interventions are paramount for improving the health of military women and must be applied when caring for this unique at-risk population.

It is the authors' recommendation that screenings begin early and occur often for military women in their childbearing years. Military women should be screened for ID to implement interventions to improve their physical fitness scores, cognitive scores, and overall well-being. The likelihood that women will be deployed to a foreign land for war or humanitarian missions is high. Waiting until women are deployed to screen is too late, because the availability of biochemical tests, such as serum ferritin, serum iron, and TIBC may be limited in austere or first-wave deployments. Therefore, it is incumbent on the military health care system to screen women for ID on an annual basis and before deployments, and provide appropriate treatment in order to put women in the best position to perform optimally to complete the military mission.

REFERENCES

1. Center for Military Readiness Policy Analysis. Why American servicewomen are serving at greater risk: women in land combat. CMR Report 2003;16:1–6. Available at: http://cmrlink.org/WomenInCombat.asp?docID=187. Accessed February 9, 2010.
2. Harrell MC, Backett MK, Chien CS, et al. The status of gender integration in the military: analysis of selected occupations. Santa Monica (CA): RAND; 2002.
3. US Census Bureau. Women history month, facts for features, CB09-FF.03. Available at: http://www.census.gov/Press-Release/www/releases/pdf/cb09ff-03.pdf. Accessed February 14, 2009.
4. Women's Research & Education Institute [WREI]. Available at: http://www.wrei. org/projects/wiu/wim/didyouknow.htm. Accessed May 13, 2009.
5. Centers for Disease Control and Prevention. Iron deficiency—United States, 1999–2000. MMWR Morb Mortal Wkly Rep 2002;51:897–9.
6. Yip R. Mineral deficiencies. In: Strickland GT, editor. Hunter's tropical medicine and emerging infectious diseases. 8th edition. Philadelphia: Saunders; 2000. p. 284–8.
7. Killip S, Bennett JM, Chambers MD. Iron deficiency anemia. Am Fam Physician 2007;75(5):671–8.
8. Institute of Medicine. Mineral requirements of military personnel: levels needed for cognitive and physical performance during garrison training. Washington, DC: National Academies Press; 2006.
9. US Department of Defense. Population representation in the military services. Available at: http://www.defenselink.mil/prhome/poprep2001/chapter2/c2_age. htm. Accessed May 13, 2009.
10. Abrams SA. Iron requirements and iron deficiency in adolescents. Available at: www.uptodate.com. Accessed September 14, 2007.
11. Beard J, Tobin B. Iron status and exercise. Am J Clin Nutr 2000;72(Suppl 2): 594S–7S.
12. Brittenham GM. Mechanisms of iron transport. In: Hoffman R, Benj E, Shattil SJ, et-al, editors. Hematology: basic principles and practice. 5th edition. Philadelphia: Churchill Livingston Elsevier; 2009. p. 453–8.

13. Wu AC, Lesperance L, Bernstein H. Screening for iron deficiency. Pediatr Rev 2002;23(5):171–8.
14. Clark SF. Iron deficiency anemia. Nutr Clin Pract 2008;23(2):128–41.
15. Heath AL, Skeaff CM, Williams S, et al. The role of blood loss and diet in the aetiology of mild iron deficiency in premenopausal adult New Zealand women. Public Health Nutr 2001;4(2):197–206.
16. Barton JC. Iron deficiency. In: Rakel RE, Bope ET, editors. Conn's current therapy 2008. 60th edition. Philadelphia: Saunders; 2008. p. 385–8.
17. Major data sources for Healthy People. 2010. Available at: http://www.healthypeople.gov/document/HTML/tracking/thp_partc.htm#NHANES. Accessed July 21, 2009.
18. Looker AC, Dallman PR, Carroll MD, et al. Prevalence of iron deficiency in the United States. JAMA 1997;277(12):973–6.
19. McClung JP, Marchitelli LJ, Friedl KE, et al. Prevalence of iron deficiency and iron deficiency anemia among three populations of female military personnel in the US Army. J Am Coll Nutr 2006;25(1):64–9.
20. Kaunitz AM. Oral contraceptive health benefits: perception versus reality. Contraception 1999;59(Suppl 1):29S–33S.
21. Cusick SE, Mei Z, Freedman DS, et al. Unexplained decline in the prevalence of anemia among US children and women between 1988–1994 and 1999–2002. Am J Clin Nutr 2008;88(6):1611–7.
22. Oh GT. Gestational diabetes among female service members in relation to body mass index prior to service, active components, US Armed Forces, 1998–2007. Med Surveill Monthly Rep 2008;15(4):2–5. Available at: http://afhsc.army.mil/viewMSMR?file=2008/v15_n04.pdf. Accessed February 9, 2010.
23. Booth CK, Coad RA, Forbes-Ewan CH, et al. The physiological and psychological effects of combat ration feeding during a 12-day training exercise in the tropics. Mil Med 2003;168(1):63–70.
24. Institute of Medicine. Dietary reference intakes (DRIs): recommended intakes for individuals. Available at: http://www.iom.edu/Object.File/Master/21/372/0.pdf. Accessed July 20, 2009.
25. Deruisseau KC, Roberts LM, Kushnick MR, et al. Iron status of young males and females performing weight-training exercise. Med Sci Sports Exerc 2004;36(2):241–8.
26. Rodenberg RE, Gustafson S. Iron as an ergogenic aid: ironclad evidence? Curr Sports Med Rep 2007;6(4):258–64.
27. Mercer KW, Densmore JJ. Hematologic disorders in the athlete. Clin Sports Med 2005;24(3):599–621, ix.
28. Hinton PS. Iron deficiency in physically active adults. ACM's Health & Fitness Journal 2006;10:12–8. Available at: http://journals.lww.com/acsm-healthfitness/toc/2006/09000. Accessed February 9, 2010.
29. Sinclair LM, Hinton PS. Prevalence of iron deficiency with and without anemia in recreationally active men and women. J Am Diet Assoc 2005;105(6):975–8.
30. Dubnov G, Foldes AJ, Mann G, et al. High prevalence of iron deficiency and anemia in female military recruits. Mil Med 2006;171(9):866–9.
31. Minares C, McGregor J, Ruth C, et al. Effect of iron supplementation on hematological adaptations to moderate altitude among former sea level females. Med Sci Sports Exerc 2009;41(5):S435.
32. Air Education and Training Command. Fighter aircrew conditioning program (AFI 11-406). Available at: http://www.usa-federal-forms.com/us-air-force-forms-pdf-optimized-version-b/aetcci11-406.pdf. Accessed July 20, 2009.

33. Vahdat Shariatpanaahi M, Vahdat Shariatpanaahi Z, Moshtaaghi M, et al. The relationship between depression and serum ferritin level. Eur J Clin Nutr 2007; 61(4):532–5.
34. Zouris JM, Wade AL, Magno CP. Injury and illness casualty distributions among US Army and Marine Corps personnel during Operational Iraqi Freedom. Mil Med 2008;173(3):247–52.
35. McClung JP, Karl JP, Cable SJ, et al. Randomized, double-blind, placebo-controlled trial of iron supplementation in female soldiers during military training: effects on iron status, physical performance, and mood. Am J Clin Nutr 2009; 90(1):124–31.
36. Rose MS, Houston CS, Fulco CS, et al. Operation Everest. II: nutrition and body composition. J Appl Physiol 1988;65(6):2545–51.
37. Brothers MD, Wilbur RL, Byrnes WC. Physical fitness and hematological changes during acclimatization to moderate altitude: a retrospective study. High Alt Med Biol 2007;8(3):213–24.
38. Brothers MD, Doan BK, Wile AL, et al. Chronic hematological and physiological adaptations following 48 weeks of moderate altitude residence. Med Sci Sports Exerc 2008;40(5):S51.
39. Brothers MD, Doan BK, Wile AL, et al. Long-term acclimatization to moderate altitude: a 4-year cross-sectional analysis. Physiologist 2008;51(6):318.
40. Bruns R, Lindsey M, Rowe K, et al. Hemoglobin drops within minutes of injuries and predicts need for an intervention to stop hemorrhage. J Trauma 2007; 63(2):312–5.
41. Brolinson PG, Elliott D. Exercise and the immune system. Clin Sports Med 2007; 26(3):311–9.
42. Cowell BS, Rosenbloom CS, Skinner R, et al. Policies on screening female athletes for iron deficiency in NCAA division I-A institutions. Int J Sport Nutr Exerc Metab 2003;13(3):277–85.
43. US Preventive Services Task Force. Screening for iron deficiency anemia. Available at: http://www.ahrq.gov/clinic/USpstf/uspsiron.htm. Accessed July 21, 2009.
44. Trego LL. Military women's menstrual experiences and interest in menstrual suppression during deployment. J Obstet Gynecol Neonatal Nurs 2007;36(4): 342–7.
45. Cogswell ME, Kettel-Khan L, Ramakrishnan U. Iron supplement use among women in the United States: science, policy, and practice. J Nutr 2003;133(6): 1974S–7S.

The Consequences of Modern Military Deployment on Calcium Status and Bone Health

Mary S. McCarthy, PhD, RN[a,b],*, Lori A. Loan, PhD, RNC[a],
Andres Azuero, PhD[c], Curtis Hobbs, MD[d]

KEYWORDS

• Bone health • Calcium • Deployment • Sweat calcium loss

The United States has been at war in Iraq and Afghanistan for more than 6 years. The Army leadership strives to ensure the safety, health, and performance of soldiers in combat. (Throughout this paper, the term "soldier" is used to refer to Army service members). However, a protracted war such as the one currently underway weakens soldiers physically and mentally. Because these soldiers return multiple times to combat areas, health care providers are keenly aware of the effect of deployment on health in general and bone health in particular.

Deployment experiences can include heavy body armor, environmental extremes, and changes in diet and exercise habits. Soldiers in Iraq and Afghanistan also experience dehydration, fatigue, and psychological stress. As a result, many military health care providers believe that deployment conditions can lead to deterioration in soldiers' physical and mental health.

This research was sponsored by the TriService Nursing Research Program (grant N06-P09), Uniformed Services University of Health Sciences; however, the information, content, or conclusions do not necessarily represent the official position or policy of, nor should any official endorsement be inferred, by the TriService Nursing Research Program, Uniformed Services of the Health Sciences, the Army Medical Department, the Department of the Army, the Department of Defense, or the US Government.
[a] Nursing Research Service, Madigan Army Medical Center, MCHJ-CN-NR, 9040A Reid Street, Tacoma, WA 98431, USA
[b] 1611 Nisqually Street, Steilacoom, WA 98388, USA
[c] Department of Nursing, University of Alabama, 1530 3rd Avenue South, Birmingham, AL 35294-1210, USA
[d] Department of Medicine, Madigan Army Medical Center, MCHJ-M, 9040A Reid Street, Tacoma, WA 98431, USA
* Corresponding author. 1611 Nisqually Street, Steilacoom, WA 98388.
E-mail address: mary.mccarthy@amedd.army.mil

Nurs Clin N Am 45 (2010) 109–122
doi:10.1016/j.cnur.2010.02.002
0029-6465/10/$ – see front matter. Published by Elsevier Inc.

By December 2009, more than 36,000 people were wounded in action, and countless others have had physical problems that can last for months or years after their overseas duty from the wear and tear of war.[1] Musculoskeletal and connective tissue disorders were the predominant illness and injury-related category for ambulatory visits in military clinics and facilities in 2008, accounting for 24% of all visits, a 15% increase from 2004.[2] The most common complaints involved the back, neck, knees, shoulders, and feet. Soldiers reported a wide range of injuries, including intervertebral disc disorders, back pain, joint disorders, and stress fractures.[2] In a 2006 report of the postdeployment health concerns of more than 118,000 returning service members,2 of 4 main health concerns of members of each military service (Army, Navy, and Air Force) were musculoskeletal.[3]

Soldiers with physical limitations are not fit and ready to be deployed, and this has a negative effect on a unit's readiness for deployment. Because of the resulting work restrictions, lost work days, and discomfort, musculoskeletal injuries have a significant effect on the health and readiness of the US Army in peacetime and in conflict.[4]

In 2006, we conducted a study to identify musculoskeletal injury data on outpatient visits of an infantry unit assigned to Fort Lewis, Washington. The unit consisted of 2329 male and female soldiers who had recently been deployed to Iraq for 12 months. The analysis of this query revealed an 11% (n = 252) incidence of fractures, dislocations, sprains, and strains. These results were consistent with those of a previous health assessment survey at this military installation.[3]

To further evaluate injuries associated with bone health, we used the Defense Medical Epidemiology Database (DMED) to identify stress fractures in soldiers aged 18 to 29 years (**Table 1**).[5] This study found approximately 20.5 stress fractures per 1000 soldiers, a substantial rate given the lost work time for medical attention and physical therapy (which involves strengthening exercises at the hospital or gym and can require absences from work for up to 2 hours 3 times a week).

In September 2008, the US Army had 1,097,050 active, National Guard, and Reserve soldiers, of whom 85% were enlisted men and women (ie, have a lower rank than commissioned officer).[6] Sixty-eight percent, or 634,095, of enlisted soldiers were between 17 and 29 years of age.[7] This age range coincides with the period of peak bone mass that occurs when the growth in the size of the bones and the accumulation of bone mineral has stabilized.[1]

Genetic factors account for 60% to 80% of peak skeletal mass, and hormonal status and environmental factors (including calcium intake and loss and weight-bearing exercise) influence the rest.[8,9]

One might expect that the physical exercise required for military occupations and the availability of high-quality dietary options in military dining facilities would place today's soldiers at low risk of poor bone health.[9] However, like other young adults, soldiers often make poor food choices when they are not deployed. These poor

Table 1 Stress fracture injury locations in soldiers aged 18 to 25 years			
ICD-9 Code	Location of Stress Fracture	Number of Injuries	Rate per 1000 Soldiers
733.93	Tibia or fibula	27	7.1
733.94	Metatarsals	8	2.11
733.95	Other bone	43	11.35

Abbreviation: ICD-9, International Classification of Diseases, 9th revision.
Source: DMED.

food choices, combined with the relaxed daily physical training requirements for nondeployed soldiers, threaten their optimal bone health.

More than a decade before the start of the Global War on Terrorism, Armstrong and colleagues[10] reported that soldiers had low calcium intake. These investigators said that soldiers could accumulate a substantial calcium deficit over time because of the combined effects of sweat loss and low dietary intake. Today, in a well-resourced war zone, evidence indicates that soldiers' dietary calcium intake is still low. Deficient calcium ingestion in an arid desert climate with an average temperature of 40 to 43°C (105–110°F) in summer months is likely to compound the effects of excessive dermal losses of calcium.[11]

Although the physical demands on soldiers vary depending on the type of work they do, every service member needs protection from the highly lethal weapons and improvised explosive devices of today's battlefield. Nonmedical Army personnel in Iraq and Afghanistan are required to wear 16 kg (35 lb) or more of personal body armor 24 hours a day, 7 days a week. This requirement is partly responsible for the unprecedented number of musculoskeletal complaints reported by service members seen in medical clinics in the combat area and on their return to the United States.[12] Furthermore, this body armor load, in conjunction with high environmental temperatures (ambient and inside heavy armored vehicles) contributes to increased sweating and accompanying dermal mineral loss, including calcium loss.

Literature on the effect of calcium lost through sweat on bone health is sparse and the few research findings available are inconclusive. Studies of basketball players and firefighters, for example, found that athletes experienced a significant decrease in bone mass density (BMD) during the basketball season but firefighters experienced no net loss of BMD during a 4-month training course.[13]

Investigators have studied the amount of calcium and other minerals lost through sweat, but these studies involved different environmental conditions than those experienced by soldiers in Iraq and Afghanistan. In 2 of these studies, the investigators measured whole-body sweat calcium concentration during exercise.[14,15] In the study conducted by Shirreffs and Maughan,[15] mean sweat calcium concentration was 52 ± 36 mg/L during exercise in a warm (34.5°C) humid environment. Costa and colleagues[16] found exercise sweat calcium concentrations of 72 ± 10 mg/L in individuals fed a space diet from NASA and 74 ± 17 mg/L in those who received a purified formula. Both groups had similar calcium intake and the study took place in a cooler (24.5°C) environment than the Shirreffs and Maughan study.[15]

The previous studies were also conducted using an assortment of collection methods that precludes generalization of the results. For example, sweat collection methods have included total body measurements and regional measurements on, for example, the back or arm. In 2 studies that compared whole-body sweat mineral content with regional measurements taken from the back or arm, higher mineral concentrations were found in the sweat from regional sites.[17,18] The investigators concluded that using regional measurements to estimate mineral losses could lead to an overestimation of total body sweat mineral losses.

Investigators have also studied sweat calcium loss using regional measurements during exercise.[13,19] Although the range of sweat calcium loss seems to be broad, the studies using regional sites and similar methodologies to collect the sweat have had similar findings. These studies found mean sweat calcium concentrations of 30 ± 5 mg/L for runners and 44 ± 12 mg/L for firefighters.[13,18]

Understanding the effect of sweat calcium loss in deployed soldiers is particularly important to nurse case managers working in military health care settings because their critical functions include keeping service members healthy and fit for duty and expediting care to return injured soldiers to their jobs. Nurse case managers are uniquely positioned to assess the effects of diet, exercise, and metabolism on the current and future health and wellness of each soldier. These nurses also coordinate specialty consultations and education to minimize long-term disability and maximize productivity in the military environment.

Several Department of Defense agencies recognize the need for further research on dietary calcium requirements for military service members during daily unit activities in the United States and during combat operations. In addition, these agencies have called for evidence supporting the link between calcium intake and bone health.

We conducted a study to help better define the links between diet, environment, and bone health in soldiers in the desert conditions that most experience in current combat environments. The study had 3 specific aims: (1) to determine the feasibility of quantifying sweat calcium loss in soldiers in a desert climate under conditions of intense physical training; (2) to examine the effect of calcium loss on short-term bone health using biochemical markers of bone formation and resorption, and dual-energy x-ray absorptiometry (DXA) to assess bone mineral quality; and (3) to describe the potential effects of self-reported exercise and dietary habits on bone health in soldiers.

METHODS
Design

The study had a prospective, descriptive, longitudinal design with repeated measures. The study took place in 2 locations in Washington State. The first location was a military training site in the Yakima desert of eastern Washington. This desert climate at this site was similar to the current combat environment, which enhanced our ability to generalize the study findings to deployed soldiers. The second location was Madigan Army Medical Center (MAMC) in Tacoma, Washington. At MAMC, data on diet, exercise, and bone mineral density were collected before and after participating soldiers were deployed to Iraq.

Participants

Fifty-two nondeploying soldiers participated in the sweat calcium data collection in the desert in September 2008. An additional 53 soldiers were recruited at MAMC where data was collected before and after their 15-month deployment in Iraq.

Study Procedures

The MAMC and Uniformed Services University of Health Sciences institutional review boards approved this study. Written informed consent was obtained from all soldiers who participated in this study.

Sweat Calcium Measurement

The commander of a male infantry unit gave us access to soldiers scheduled for training in the Yakima desert. The sweat collection method was adapted from procedures used at the University of Texas at Houston and endorsed by the Gatorade Institute (Ed Coyle, PhD, Houston, TX, USA, and Craig Horswill, PhD, Gainesville, FL, USA, personal communication, January 2007).

We collected data on 2 occasions, 1 week apart in September 2008. Temperatures ranged from 6°C in the morning to 29°C by 2 PM.

During these data-collection visits, research team members were dressed in civilian attire with no evidence of rank or position to avoid any suggestion of coercion. At the start of the first visit, the principal investigator (PI) briefly explained the study procedures and asked for volunteers to have their sweat calcium level measured. Volunteers signed a consent form.

The PI checked all consent forms for completeness, measured the height and weight of volunteers, restocked supplies, and answered questions from participants.

For the sweat collection, soldiers assembled in the unit area wearing the Army physical training uniform consisting of shorts and a tee shirt. The research team collected sweat samples between 6:00 AM and 8:00 AM; the temperature was between 6 and 10°C.

The PI chose the type of sweat patch used in this study to collect sweat samples for analysis after discussions with many experts at research centers around the United States. The patch that most investigators recommended was no longer available. However, the research team used an alternate patch with much success, although the technique needs refinement because a large volume of the sweat sample was lost if the patch became unsecured. Experts warned of a 20% failure rate, which was one reason for using 2 sweat patches (on the arm and back) on each soldier.

Study personnel first cleaned the arm and back sites chosen for the sweat patch applications with distilled water. Gauze sponges were then affixed to the skin of one upper arm and the right lower back and the sponges were secured with Tegaderm (3M, St Paul, MN, USA) clear film after using Skin Prep (Smith & Nephew, London, UK) to promote adherence to the skin. The soldiers were then instructed to perform vigorous exercise for 30 to 45 minutes under the guidance of the senior ranking soldier in each group; each senior ranking solder was given a stopwatch to monitor the length of the exercise period. Most soldiers participated in group physical training for 35 minutes.

Individual 0.5-L bottles of water containing no added calcium were available to participants for hydration during exercise. The soldiers kept track of the number of bottles of water they consumed during the exercise period to enable the team to accurately calculate their sweat rate.

After exercising, all soldiers returned to the unit area to have their sweat patches removed by research team members. Immediately after removing the saturated gauze sponges, they were placed in 60-mL syringes. Depressing the syringe barrel forced the sweat sample through a filter into a 15-mL test tube. The specimens were augmented with 10 mL of distilled water for optimal extraction later and the test tubes were capped for transportation and storage. The sweat specimens were placed in a Coleman cooler overnight and the cooler was delivered to the laboratory at MAMC the following day. At MAMC, the samples were placed in a freezer at −57°C until the analysis was performed.

Some of the soldiers who contributed sweat samples also volunteered to provide a complete-void urine specimen so that the study team could calculate total body sweat rate; these calculations also required height and weight measurements to adjust for body surface area. Vertical height was measured to the nearest 0.1 cm using a portable stadiometer (Seca, Terre Haute, IN, USA) and weight was measured using a lightweight prezeroed digital scale that accommodated up to 181 kg (Detecto, Youngstown, OH, USA). All other soldiers provided a spot-void urine specimen for calcium analysis.

Urine specimens were placed in Ziplock bags, each bag coded with the participant's identification number, and the bags were packed on ice in a second Coleman cooler for transport to MAMC. Because sweat calcium measurement is not a routine clinical test, the PI conducted the analyses in the clinical investigations laboratory (author MM) using the Quantitative Colorimetric Calcium Assay Kit (BioAssay Systems, Hayward, CA, USA). The PI conducted all tests twice and a senior molecular biologist provided quality control supervision for the analysis. Standard curve plots for individual analyses were all within an acceptable range.

Diet, Exercise, and BMD Data Collection

For the diet, exercise, and BMD phase of this study, the commander of a noninfantry unit that was preparing to deploy gave permission for the PI to solicit male and female volunteers. Soldier volunteers consented to complete diet and exercise questionnaires, have blood drawn to assess bone turnover, and undergo DXA to assess bone mineral density. These volunteers completed the predeployment data collection at the hospital outpatient clinic. At MAMC, 3 stations were set up for data collection: one for completing the questionnaires, one for the DXA procedure, and one for a brief physical examination by a nurse practitioner. Soldiers were instructed to go to the laboratory to have their blood drawn in between the other stations.

The soldiers completed the Block Food Frequency Questionnaire (FFQ, Nutrition-Quest, Berkeley, CA, USA) twice, once before their deployment to Iraq and once on their return. The FFQ solicits recall for the previous year, asking questions such as "In the past year, how many times did you drink milk?" Answer choices for this question are "once a day, once a week, once a month, or more frequently." The FFQ captures information on food eaten at home, in restaurants, or as take-out, and it is sensitive to different cultural preferences.[20] NutritionQuest conducted a comprehensive nutrient analysis of foods and supplements that soldiers reported in their FFQ responses and prepared a report on the dietary intake of each participating soldier.

The study used the Baecke Habitual Physical Activity Questionnaire (the Netherlands) to assess physical activity during work, sports, and leisure. Each occupation is coded by the level of physical work involved. The work and leisure subscales are scored from 1 to 5, with 1 for never and 5 for always/very often. The sport score was determined by assigning values to the sports according to their intensity, the amount of time spent doing the sport, and frequency of the activity. A formula was then applied to calculate the final physical activity score.[21]

Soldiers presented to the MAMC Department of Nuclear Medicine for the DXA scan (Prodigy, Lunar Corp, Madison, WI, USA) wearing Army physical training clothes. A dedicated DXA technician performed the scans. The DXA scan involved lumbar spine and femur readings; outputs included T score, Z score, and BMD. The T score compares the individual's BMD in standard deviations with the average peak BMD in healthy young adults.[22] The Z score compares the individual's BMD with the mean BMD of persons in the same age group.[22] Age and ethnicity are considered in these comparisons; female gender, low body mass index (BMI, calculated as weight in kilograms divided by the square of height in meters), tobacco use, high bone turnover rates, and family history of osteoporosis all contribute to a higher risk of osteoporosis.[23]

During the physical examination, the soldiers underwent a body composition assessment that included measurements of height in inches using a Harpenden stadiometer, weight in pounds using an electronic scale, BMI, and waist circumference using a plastic-coated tape at the minimal abdominal circumference (women) or the navel level (men) rounded down to the nearest 0.5 in.[24] The physical examination also included a body fat-water analysis using near-infrared reactance (NIR) technology (Futrex, Inc, Hagerstown, MD, USA). During the physical examination, the practitioner documented the soldier's family history of bone disease; endocrine or eating disorder; menstrual irregularities; and alcohol, tobacco, or dietary supplement use, including use of vitamins, minerals, and body-building protein powder. Participants received a copy of their body composition report and study personnel educated them about

YEAR ALL HOST ANG NESTOM

their optimal body weight, BMI, and hydration if their NIR analysis results indicated low hydration status.

The bone health indices measured before deployment included osteocalcin for bone turnover, bone-specific alkaline phosphatase level for bone formation, tartrate-resistant acid phosphatase (TRAP) level for bone resorption, total calcium level, or some combination of these indices (**Table 2**). Postdeployment indices measured were the same as before deployment, and carboxyterminal telopeptide, a marker of bone resorption, and insulin-like growth factor-1 (IGF-1), an endocrine marker, were also measured. Because the TRAP analysis was technically cumbersome, this test was not done after deployment. Serum calcium levels were measured before and after deployment and vitamin D levels after deployment.

On completion of predeployment data collection, each participant received a $25 gift card for the Army's retail services.

The PI maintained e-mail contact with unit leaders and a few soldiers throughout the soldiers' deployment period to sustain a connection that would facilitate postdeployment data collection. On return from deployment, participants underwent the bone health tests. After completing these procedures, participants again received a gift card.

RESULTS
Demographic Characteristics

The study sample consisted of 105 soldiers assigned to Fort Lewis, Washington, from August 2007 to May 2009. This sample included 52 male soldiers who participated in the sweat calcium assessment and did not deploy to Iraq, and 53 male and female soldiers who did deploy to Baghdad, Iraq, and completed diet, exercise, and BMD assessments before their deployment. Twenty-seven percent (n = 14) of the soldiers in the sweat collection study voluntarily provided a complete-void urine specimen; the remaining 73% (n = 38) provided a spot-void urine specimen. Eighteen of the soldiers who deployed to Iraq returned for follow-up data collection.

Age was the only demographic variable recorded for soldiers participating in the sweat collection; their mean age was 25.1 years (range 19–39 years).

The demographic characteristics of the 53 volunteers who participated in the pre- and postdeployment data collection are presented in **Table 3**. Thirty-two percent of these soldiers (n = 17) reported tobacco use at baseline; several more soldiers began smoking and some who already smoked began smoking more cigarettes each day during deployment. Before deployment, 53% of participants in the pre- and postdeployment data collection reported alcohol use, with 32% (n = 17) admitting to

Table 2
Bone turnover marker levels in male and women soldiers before and after deployment to Iraq: pre- and postdeployment study (N = 53)

| | | Before Deployment | | | After Deployment | | | |
| | | Men | | Women | | Men | | Women |
	n	Mean (SD)	n	Mean (SD)	n	Mean (SD)	n	Mean (SD)
Calcium (mg/dL)	43	9.4 (0.3)	22	9.7 (0.3)	15	9.74(0.29)	7	9.57(0.35)
Vitamin D (ng/L)					10	25.5. (3.3)	5	39.4 (7.9)
BS alkaline phosphatase (μg/L)	10	16.8 (3.1)	5	11.3 (4.8)	11	17.6 (4.9)	7	11.5 (4.3)
Osteocalcin (ng/L)	10	26.6 (6.1)	5	19 (9.3)	11	13.1 (4.4)	7	17.6 (9.3)
TRAP (U/L)	29	4.78 (1.32)	19	4.78(1.10)	4	4.35 (1.32)	5	4.12 (0.63)

WESTERN IOWA TECH-LIBRARY

Table 3
Demographic characteristics of deploying soldiers: pre- and postdeployment study (N = 53)

Characteristic	
Age in years, mean (SD)	23.1 (3.9)
Female gender, n (%)	19 (35.8)
Ethnicity[a] n (%)	
Caucasian	26 (50.0)
African American	13 (25.0)
Hispanic	9 (17.3)
Asian	2 (3.9)
Pacific Islander	1 (1.9)
Other	1 (1.9)
Rank, n (%)	
Officer	4 (7.6)
Enlisted	49 (92.4)

[a] One missing observation.

consuming at least 3 drinks a week and 11.3% consuming up to 12 drinks a week. Alcohol consumption was prohibited during the deployment period.

Twenty-nine percent (n = 5) of female soldiers reported using oral contraceptives before deployment and none of the women reported amenorrhea. A urine human chorionic gonadotropin test was ordered for all women to determine their pregnancy status. Pregnancy was confirmed in 1 woman; she was ineligible for deployment and for continuation in the study. Another female soldier became pregnant during her deployment and returned to Fort Lewis; she did not return for study follow-up. Forty-three percent (n = 3) of the 7 female soldiers who returned for follow-up reported taking oral contraceptives or other estrogen treatment for birth control.

Weight and BMI

The mean BMI (25.9 kg/m^2) of male soldiers in this study exceeded the acceptable BMI standard of 24.9 kg/m^2 before deployment and was essentially unchanged when the soldiers returned from deployment (**Table 4**). The mean BMI of female soldiers was within the normal range before and after deployment. However, some women's weight increased by up to 10 lb, their body fat increased by up to 2%, and their waist circumference grew by 2 inches by the time they returned from deployment.

Sweat Calcium Loss

The normal range of sweat calcium is 16 to 88 mg/L.[17] Based on the standardized formula we used to calculate calcium losses, most soldiers in this study experienced normal sweat calcium losses (n = 47, mean [M] = 59.2 mg/L, standard deviation [SD] = 29.5 mg/L), yet 18% had losses that exceeded the normal range (n = 5, M = 111.2 mg/L, SD = 9.5 mg/L) (**Table 5**).

Impact of Calcium Deficits on Bone Health

During their 15 months of deployment, soldiers maintained calcium homeostasis, with a narrow range for normal values of 8.4 to 10.2 mg/dL.

Normal vitamin D levels are 30 to 100 ng (ng)/L; levels lower than 30 ng/L indicate vitamin D insufficiency and people with levels lower than 20 ng/L require treatment.

WESTERN IOWA TECH-LIBRARY

Table 4
Anthropometric characteristics of soldiers: pre- and postdeployment study (N=53)

	Before Deployment				After Deployment			
	Men		Women		Men		Women	
	n	Mean (SD)	n	Mean (SD)	n	Mean (SD)	n	Mean (SD)
Height (in)	32	70.1 (2.9)	19	64.7 (3.2)				
Weight (lb)	32	181.2 (27.4)	19	142.9 (25.3)	14	177.2 (23.4)	7	135.6 (9.6)
BMI (kg/m²)	32	25.9 (3.4)	19	23.9 (3.1)	14	25.1 (3.6)	7	24 (2.1)
Body fat (%)	35	15.9 (4.4)	14	26.9 (4.7)	13	14 (6.5)	7	27.6 (3.5)
Waist circumference (inches)	35	34.3 (4.2)	13	28.8 (3.9)	14	31.6 (3.1)	7	29.3 (2.3)

The range of values for participating soldiers was 7 to 71 ng/mL, with only 3 of 18 soldiers having a vitamin D level higher than 30 ng/mL.

The expected range for changes in BMD of the femur over 15 months is ±2% for individuals aged 19 to 39 years. In this study, 6 of 18 (33%) participants had a BMD after deployment that was more than 2% lower than that shown by their initial DXA, but 1 participant's femur bone mass increased by 2.1% (**Table 6**). The expected range for changes in BMD of the lumbar spine is ±1% in this age category. Here too, findings were mixed, with decreases in lumbar spine BMD in 3 of 18 (17%) participants exceeding the expected 1% at postdeployment follow-up, suggesting bone loss. Conversely, lumbar spine BMD increased by more than 1% in 7 participants.

Effect of Exercise and Diet on Deployed Soldiers' Bone Health

Results for self-reported exercise are provided in **Table 7**. In general, exercise levels from work, sports, and leisure activities were similar before and after deployment.

DISCUSSION

The process of quantifying sweat calcium loss was feasible but logistically challenging. The amounts of calcium lost by soldiers in the current study (59.2 ± 29.5 mg/dL) are similar to those reported by previous investigators using a similar methodology.[19] The intensity of the exercise and its short duration in this study make it difficult to estimate dermal calcium losses over a lengthy deployment when soldiers are wearing military uniforms, body armor, backpacks, water containers, and helmets in at least 30°C heat. It is apparent that a subset of soldiers in any unit may be at high risk of excessive calcium losses with uncertain consequences on bone health.

Although acclimatization occurs over time in any environment, not all minerals are affected equally. Studies suggest that although sweat calcium losses decrease with acclimatization to heat, urinary calcium losses do not change over time.[25] A larger sample of soldiers is needed to perform the definitive research necessary to advise

Table 5
Calcium losses in soldiers: sweat patch study (N = 52)

	Sweat Calcium Level (mg/L)	Sweat Rate (L/h)	Urine Calcium Level (mg/L)
Mean level	59.2 ± 29.5	1.2 ± 0.67	100.9 ± 0.6
Range	6–119	0–2.4 (fluid loss)	<10.0–290.8
Normal range	16–88	Up to 2	≤220 mg/L

Table 6
Bone health of soldiers: pre- and postdeployment study (N = 53)

	Predeployment Level, Mean (SD) (n = 52)	Postdeployment Level, Mean (SD) (n = 18)
Femur BMD	1.15 (0.15)	1.1 (0.12)
Femur DXA, T score	0.6 (1)	0.3 (0.9)
Spine BMD	25 (0.12)	1.25 (0.12)
Spine DXA, t score	0.4 (1)	0.3 (1)

military commanders and health care professionals about the hazards of prolonged combat duty in a desert climate and its effect on mineral losses and bone health.

In general, the participants had normal bone turnover based on osteocalcin and TRAP results, although 10% (n = 5) of participants had lower than normal and 10% had higher than normal bone turnover rates at baseline. The differences in bone turnover rates could have been because of age differences among participants, with more rapid turnover occurring in younger soldiers. We plan to conduct further analyses to evaluate the associations between age, ethnicity, gender, endocrine status, alcohol and tobacco use, and bone turnover.

IGF-1 levels were assessed as a result of reports in the literature that prolonged periods of stress can negatively affect bone metabolism by increasing bone resorption; this can be identified by a decrease in levels of IGF-1. This biomarker is also useful for evaluating nutritional stress; underfeeding and protein-calorie deficits result in substantial reductions in IGF-1 concentration.[26] The normal IGF-1 concentration is 126 to 382 ng/mL; no soldier in the study had deficient or excess IGF-1 levels before or after deployment. Because of the high cost of bone turnover marker assessments and their lack of sufficient sensitivity and specificity to predict stress fracture risk, we recommend that investigators select the minimum number of tests needed to measure bone formation, bone resorption, and bone turnover for use in conjunction with DXA.[26]

Vitamin D deficiency is now recognized as a widespread problem in many countries, including the United States.[27] The major source of vitamin D for most adults is sunlight exposure. Other sources include oily fish and fortified foods such as milk, cereals, and bread. The soldiers in this study met the minimum requirement for daily vitamin D intake of 200 IU for adults up to 50 years of age, but they were able to achieve this only by consuming supplemental vitamin D (see **Table 2**). The soldiers in this study were probably exposed to some sunlight during their deployment in a hot desert location, so one possible explanation for the low levels of vitamin D in this sample is the lack of dietary intake from fortified foods. Soldiers reported they did not consume large quantities of milk in Baghdad because of its unpleasant taste. Increased skin pigmentation, obesity, and the application of sunscreen also limit production of vitamin D and

Table 7
Baecke physical activity indices: pre- and postdeployment study (N=53)

Index	Before Deployment		After Deployment	
	n	Mean (SD)	n	Mean (SD)
Work	48	3.1 (0.5)	18	3 (0.4)
Sport	43	3.7 (1.2)	18	4.1 (1.5)
Leisure	48	2.8 (0.5)	19	3 (0.7)

could help explain the low vitamin D levels in this sample.[27] One study in Hawaii found that vitamin D levels in adults were lower than 30 ng/mL, despite an average of 15 hours per week of sun exposure over 3 months, providing further evidence that sunlight alone is not sufficient to maintain adequate vitamin D stores.[28]

BMD is the most predictive measure of fracture risk.[26] The Department of Defense has examined strategies for improving the bone health of service members, with a focus on decreasing the incidence of stress fractures during intense physical training and reducing the risk of osteoporosis.[29] The department's research efforts have been primarily directed at ways to prevent stress fractures in new military recruits. Despite these efforts, the number of stress fracture injuries over the past few years has increased among soldiers returning from lengthy deployments. Stress fractures are a particular concern in the combat environment, where soldiers are less likely to seek medical attention for an injury perceived as minor and the medical equipment needed for proper diagnosis might not be readily available. Furthermore, it has been shown that nonsteroidal antiinflammatory medications could slow down stress fracture healing.[30]

The individual nutrient profiles showed that many study participants had a calcium deficit although, on average, the soldiers participating in the study were able to just meet or minimally exceed the military dietary reference intake (DRI) for calcium before and after deployment. The current military DRI and reference intake for garrison training (intense training and 1-day missions) for calcium is 1000 mg a day for men and women, the same as the Institute of Medicine's DRI.[31] Military experts have questioned whether this intake level is sufficient for optimal performance of military duties, given the potential for excessive losses of calcium. The soldiers in this study reported that food in Iraq was plentiful and flavorful, with large serving sizes and no restrictions on second helpings.

The war in most areas of Iraq is fought from solid, functional, urban structures with abundant recreational facilities such as gymnasiums, basketball courts, and pools nearby. However, soldiers also have access to fast-food restaurants and all-you-can-eat dining facilities. When questioned, many soldiers in this study did not report participating in sports or physical activities during deployment that involved weight-bearing or resistance, activities that are most beneficial to bone health. To ensure optimal BMD and reduce their risk of musculoskeletal injury, soldiers clearly need assistance in making healthy diet choices and encouragement to adopt a lifestyle that includes more vigorous physical activity.

SUMMARY

Maintaining a fit and ready force is critical to this nation's defense and this requires physical fitness.[24,32] The multitude of factors contributing to high bone turnover in the deployed environment, including stress, substantial sweat calcium losses, changes in diet and physical activity, body armor weight, and smoking, make all deployed soldiers vulnerable to musculoskeletal injuries and stress fractures. These injuries can affect bone health in later years for all soldiers, but especially those who are injured before they have achieved peak bone mass.

The most important modifiable risk factors associated with bone health include hormonal status, physical activity, and nutrition.[33–35] Health promotion for all military personnel must focus on education about the role of nutrition and exercise in developing and maintaining strong bones. Such health promotion initiatives should target soldiers between the ages of 19 and 30 years because they have not yet achieved peak bone mass. With each soldier encounter, military nurses are in a position to reinforce the importance of a healthy diet and regular weight-bearing exercise to promote strong bones.

Key areas of ongoing investigation include determining the dose of vitamin D necessary to maintain healthy levels in all military personnel, evaluating the influence of nutritional status on bone health, and examining the role of vitamin and mineral supplements on bone quality.[29] Future studies need to identify the most clinically useful bone health biomarkers, interventions that promote healthy nutrition and exercise in military service members, and strategies to minimize injury during military training and combat duty.

In this article, the authors highlight the potentially negative effect of the current combat environment on the bone health of young military men and women. These soldiers could be at risk of stress fractures and future bone disease as a result of an unhealthy diet and low physical activity levels during deployment. The authors examined a combination of physiologic biomarkers, including bone turnover and bone mineral density, and nutrition and exercise surveys to collect data on potential bone health risks related to deployment. Soldiers participating in the investigation of bone health before and after deployment did not have decreased bone density but the study did raise awareness of an issue that might otherwise go unnoticed as preventive care is typically focused on older adults. Several risk factors for musculoskeletal injury during deployment might be modifiable. Nurses have the necessary skills for counseling and monitoring behaviors that can minimize the risk of disabling musculoskeletal injuries that affect quality of life and unit readiness.

REFERENCES

1. Operation Iraqi Freedom (OIF)/Operation Enduring Freedom (OEF) US Casualty Status. 7 December 2009, US Department of Defense. Defense link casualty report 2009. Available at: www.defense.gov/news/casualty.pdf. Accessed December 7, 2009.
2. Armed Forces Health Surveillance Center. Ambulatory visits among members of active components, U.S. Armed Forces, 2008. MSMR 2009;16:10–5.
3. Armed Forces Health Surveillance Center. Post-Deployment Health Reassessment (PDHRA) Program, U.S. Armed Forces: responses by service and component, September 2005-August 2006. MSMR 2006;12:2–13.
4. Jennings BM, Yoder LH, Heiner SL, et al. Soldiers with musculoskeletal injuries. J Nurs Scholarsh 2008;40:268–74.
5. Armed Forces Health Surveillance Center. Defense medical epidemiology Database. Available at: http://afhsc.mil. Accessed February 9, 2010.
6. Department of the Army Deputy Chief of Staff of Personnel. Army demographics, FY08 Army profile. Available at: http://www.armyg1.army.mil/hr/demographics.asp. Accessed February 9, 2010.
7. Department of the Army Deputy Chief of Staff of Personnel. Army demographics: FY06 army profile. Available at: http://www.armyg1.army.mil/hr/demographics.asp. Accessed February 9, 2010.
8. Kerstetter JE, O'Brien KO, Insogna KL. Dietary protein, calcium metabolism, and skeletal homeostasis revisited. Am J Clin Nutr 2003;78:584S–92S.
9. Slemenda CW, Miller JZ, Hui SL, et al. Role of physical activity in the development of skeletal mass in children. J Bone Miner Res 1991;6:1227–33.
10. Armstrong LE, Szlyk PC, De Luca JP, et al. Fluid-electrolyte losses in uniforms during prolonged exercise at 30 degrees C. Aviat Space Environ Med 1992;63:351–5.

11. National Oceanic and Atmospheric Administration. NOAA's climate summaries for the Middle East and Iraq. 2003. Available at: http://www.magazine.noaa. gov/stories/mag87.htm. Accessed February 9, 2010.
12. Konitzer LN, Fargo MV, Brininger TL, et al. Association between back, neck, and upper extremity musculoskeletal pain and the individual body armor. J Hand Ther 2008;21(2):143–8.
13. O'Toole ML, Johnson KC, Satterfield S, et al. Do sweat calcium losses affect bone mass during firefighter training? J Occup Environ Med 2000;42:1054–9.
14. Palacios C, Wigertz K, Weaver CM. Comparison of 24 hour whole body versus patch tests for estimating body surface electrolyte losses. Int J Sport Nutr Exerc Metab 2003;13:479–88.
15. Shirreffs SM, Maughan RJ. Whole body sweat collection in humans: an improved method with preliminary data on electrolyte content. J Appl Physiol 1997;82: 336–41.
16. Costa F, Calloway DH, Margen S. Regional and total body sweat composition of men fed controlled diets. Am J Clin Nutr 1969;22:52–8.
17. Jacob RA, Sandstead HH, Munoz JM, et al. Whole body surface loss of trace metals in normal males. Am J Clin Nutr 1981;34:1379–83.
18. Klesges RC, Ward KD, Shelton ML, et al. Changes in bone mineral content in male athletes. Mechanisms of action and intervention effects. JAMA 1996;276: 226–30.
19. Bullen DB, O'Toole ML, Johnson KC. Calcium losses resulting from an acute bout of moderate-intensity exercise. Int J Sport Nutr 1999;9:275–84.
20. Block G, Woods M, Potosky A, et al. Validation of a self-administered diet history questionnaire using multiple diet records. J Clin Epidemiol 1990;43: 1327–35.
21. Baecke JA, Burema J, Frijters JE. A short questionnaire for the measurement of habitual physical activity in epidemiological studies. Am J Clin Nutr 1982;36: 936–42.
22. Brunader R, Shelton DK. Radiologic bone assessment in the evaluation of osteoporosis. Am Fam Physician 2002;65:1357–64.
23. National Institutes of Health. Osteoporosis prevention, diagnosis, and therapy. NIH Consens Statement 2000;17:1–36.
24. Department of the Army. Army Regulation 600–9: the Army Weight Control Program. Washington, DC: Department of the Army; 2006.
25. Consolazio CF, Matoush LO, Nelson RA, et al. Relationship between calcium in sweat, calcium balance, and calcium requirements. J Nutr 1962;78:78–88.
26. Committee on Metabolic Monitoring for Military Field Applications SCoMNR. Monitoring metabolic status: predicting decrements in physiological and cognitive performance. Washington, DC: Food and Nutrition Board, Institute of Medicine; 2004.
27. Holick MF. The vitamin D epidemic and its health consequences. J Nutr 2005;135: 2739S–48S.
28. Binkley N, Novotny R, Krueger D, et al. Low vitamin D status despite abundant sun exposure. J Clin Endocrinol Metab 2007;92:2130–5.
29. Military Operational Medicine Research Program. Bone health and military medical readiness (BHMMR). Available at: https://momrp.amedd.army.mil/ bone_health_index.html. Accessed February 9, 2010.
30. Evans RK, Antczak AJ, Lester M, et al. Effects of a 4-month recruit training program on markers of bone metabolism. Med Sci Sports Exerc 2008;40: S660–70.

31. Committee on Mineral Requirements for Cognitive and Physical Performance of Military Personnel CoMNR. Mineral requirements for military personnel: levels needed for cognitive and physical performance during garrison training. Washington, DC: Food and Nutrition Board, Institute of Medicine; 2006.
32. Potter RN, Gardner JW, Deuster PA, et al. Musculoskeletal injuries in an Army airborne population. Mil Med 2002;167:1033–40.
33. Sambrook P, Kelly P, Eisman J. Bone mass and ageing. Baillieres Clin Rheumatol 1993;7:445–57.
34. Krall EA, Dawson-Hughes B. Heritable and life-style determinants of bone mineral density. J Bone Miner Res 1993;8:1–9.
35. Kelly PJ, Eisman JA. Osteoporosis: genetic effects on bone turnover and bone density. Ann Med 1993;25:99–101.

US Public Health Service Commissioned Corps Nurses: Responding in Times of National Need

Annette Tyree Debisette, PhD, RN[a],*,
Angela M. Martinelli, PhD, RN, CNOR[b],
Mary Pat Couig, MPH, RN[c], Michelle Braun, MSN, CRNP[d]

KEYWORDS

- US Public Health Service • Emergency preparedness
- Disaster response • Public health service nursing
- Commissioned Corps

THE US PUBLIC HEALTH SERVICE

The overarching mission of the Commissioned Corps of the US Public Health Service (PHS) is to protect, promote, and advance the health and safety of the nation. The Corps comprises more than 6400 active-duty public health professionals who develop and implement a broad range of public health programs. Being one of America's 7 uniformed services (**Box 1**), it fills essential public health leadership and service roles within major federal agencies and programs. The Corps is a vital component of the PHS, the largest public health program in the world.[1] This article presents an overview of the PHS and how Commissioned Corps officers respond during times of national and global need.

Disclaimer: The views expressed in this article do not necessarily represent the views of the US Department of Health and Human Services, US Public Health Service, Food and Drug Administration, or the National Institutes of Health or the US government.

[a] US Public Health Service, Food and Drug Administration, Office of Regulatory Affairs, Division of Human Resource Development, 11919 Rockville Pike, Rockville, MD 20852, USA
[b] Division of Treatment and Recovery Research, National Institute on Alcohol Abuse and Alcoholism, Room 2038, 5635 Fishers Lane, Rockville, MD 20852, USA
[c] US Public Health Service, 7106 Oakridge Avenue, Chevy Chase, Bethesda, MD 20815, USA
[d] US Public Health Service, Kidney Disease Section, National Institutes of Health, Clinical Center, 10 Center Drive, CRC/5-2551, Bethesda, MD 20892, USA
* Corresponding author. US Public Health Service, Food and Drug Administration, Office of Regulatory Affairs, Division of Human Resource Development, 11919 Rockville Pike, Rockville, MD 20852.
E-mail address: Annette.debisette@fda.hhs.gov

Nurs Clin N Am 45 (2010) 123–135
doi:10.1016/j.cnur.2010.02.003
0029-6465/10/$ – see front matter. Published by Elsevier Inc.

nursing.theclinics.com

> **Box 1**
> **The 7 uniformed services of the United States[a]**
>
> - US Army (1775) (Department of Defense)
> - US Marine Corps (1775) (Department of Defense)
> - US Navy (1775) (Department of Defense)
> - US Coast Guard (1790) (Department of Defense)
> - US Public Health Service (1798) (Department of Health and Human Services)
> - National Oceanic and Atmospheric Administration (1807) (Department of Commerce)
> - US Air Force (1947) (Department of Defense)
>
> [a] Based on chronology of founding.

A Historical Overview of the PHS and the Commissioned Corps

Like other uniformed services, the PHS has a long and impressive history. The federal focus on public health began in 1798 when an act of the Fifth Congress of the United States established the Marine Hospital Service (1798–1902), whose purpose was to provide health care for sick and diseased seamen.[2] In 1870, it was reorganized by combining all its hospitals under a centralized administration headquartered in Washington, DC. John Maynard Woodworth was appointed as the first supervising surgeon of the Marine Hospital Service; this position later became the US Surgeon General. Woodworth adopted a military model for his physicians, requiring them to wear uniforms and pass examinations.

In 1889, the Commissioned Corps was officially authorized, and initially only medical officers were permitted to join; later it was expanded to allow the admission of other health professionals. The officers were given the same titles and pay as officers in other uniformed services, in accordance with the US Army and US Navy pay scales. The Marine Hospital Service evolved into the Public Health and Marine Hospital Service (1902–1912), and the official name was changed to Public Health Service in 1912.[3]

PHS Commissioned Corps Nurse Category

The Public Health Services Act of 1944 authorized the commissioning of nurses and other health care professionals to the Corps.[2] Restructuring of the PHS in 1949 created the position of Chief Nurse Officer (CNO) with the rank of Assistant Surgeon General (Rear Admiral) in the Office of the Surgeon General (OSG). Lucile Petry Leone became the first nurse to serve in this position and the first woman to achieve flag rank in the PHS or in any other uniformed services of the United States.[4] In addition to serving as the chief professional officer for the nurse category, the CNO, at present, provides advice to and works with the US Surgeon General on policy issues related to nursing and public health and represents the OSG and the PHS at groups at the state, national, and international levels and at professional societies concerned with these areas.

The different health professions are organized into sections called "categories." The nurse category is the largest in the Commissioned Corps. As of July 9, 2009, there were 1504 Corps nurse officers holding positions in the United States and abroad. Most of them are assigned to operating divisions within the Department of Health and Human Services (DHHS); the rest are detailed to other federal agencies (non-DHHS). The DHHS and non-DHHS agencies, descriptions of the nurses' duties, and the number of nurses assigned are outlined in **Box 2** and in **Table 1**. Nurse officers provide direct care or perform administrative duties. For example, they provide direct clinical care in the Indian Health Service (IHS) and community health centers, the Department of Justice's Federal Bureau of Prisons (BOP), and US Marshals Service and the Department of Homeland Security's Division of Immigration Health Services. About 30% of PHS nurses have previous military experience. They transfer from other uniformed services, such as the Army or Navy, through a mechanism known as an "interservice transfer."

To qualify as an officer in the Corps, PHS nurses must have at least a baccalaureate degree in nursing. Unlike the military services, the PHS has no enlisted members. Career progression is encouraged. To be competitive for promotion to higher ranks, nurse officers are advised to pursue advanced degrees and training in nursing or health-related disciplines, such as public health.

THE NATION'S HEALTH DEPARTMENT

"The Department of Health and Human Services is the US federal government's principal agency for protecting America's health by providing essential human services, especially to those Americans who are least able to help themselves."[1]

The PHS is the primary division of the DHHS. The DHHS consists of the Office of the Secretary, staff offices, and 11 operating divisions (also known as agencies). Staff offices and operating divisions report directly to the secretary for health and human services. The DHHS includes approximately 300 programs, covering a wide spectrum of public health and science activities, such as health and social science research to prevent disease and to assure food and drug safety, and the Medicare and Medicaid programs. Most nurses are assigned to the operating divisions. In addition, the DHHS is responsible for medical preparedness for emergencies, including potential terrorist attacks.

Box 2
Examples of Commissioned Corps nurses' duties

- Perform traditional clinical services, including inpatient and outpatient care, ranging from newborn care to geriatric services, from obstetrics to orthopedics, from prevention services to chronic disease care or acute disease management

- Conduct research

- Manage the review and approval of drugs and medical products

- Respond to public health emergencies

- Develop and implement national health policies

- Develop and implement clinical practice guidelines and evidence-based reports on health care

- Coordinate prevention and education efforts on various public health issues

- Develop nursing training and education programs for basic and advanced practice nurses

- In some assignments, the focus is on improving clinical care for an entire community of patients. Although there is plenty of direct patient care, there are opportunities to work on organized national disease prevention and health promotion programs that can make an impact on disease rates, health disparities, and lives of individual patients

Table 1
DHHS and non-DHHS operating divisions, their foci, and number of nurses assigned

Name of DHHS Agency (Number of Nurses Assigned)	Agency Mission	Name of Non-DHHS Agency (Number of Nurses Assigned)	Agency Mission
Administration of Children and Families (ACF) (3)	The ACF within the DHHS is responsible for federal programs that promote the economic and social well-being of families, children, individuals, and communities	Federal Bureau of Prisons (BOP) (291)	The BOP is responsible for the custody and care of more than 204,000 federal offenders Approximately 82% of these inmates are confined in its operated facilities, whereas the remaining are confined in secure, privately managed or community-based facilities and local jails
Agency for Healthcare Research and Quality (AHRQ) (3)	AHRQ's mission is to improve the quality, safety, efficiency, and effectiveness of health care for all Americans Information from AHRQ's research helps people make informed decisions and improve the quality of health care services. AHRQ was formerly known as the Agency for Health Care Policy and Research	Department of Homeland Security (DHS) (190)	The DHS's overriding and urgent mission is to lead the unified national effort to secure the country and preserve our freedom
Agency for Toxic Substances and Disease Registry (ATSDR) (3)	The ATSDR serves the public by using the best science, taking responsive public health actions, and providing trusted information to prevent harmful exposures and diseases related to toxic substances	Department of Defense (DOD) (10)	The DOD, which includes the Army, Navy, Marines, Coast Guard, and Air Force, serves to protect and defend the citizens and the Constitution of the United States
Centers for Disease Control and Prevention (CDC) (48)	The CDC collaborates to create the expertise, information, and tools that people and communities need to protect their health—through health promotion; prevention of disease, injury, and disability; and preparedness for new health threats	Environmental Protection Agency (EPA) (1)	EPA leads the nation's environmental science, research, education, and assessment efforts. Its mission is to protect human health and the environment. Since 1970, EPA has been working for a cleaner, healthier environment for the American people

Agency	Description
Centers for Medicare and Medicaid Services (CMS) (47)	The mission of the CMS is to ensure effective, up-to-date health care coverage and to promote quality care for beneficiaries
Food and Drug Administration (FDA) (141)	The FDA protects consumers and enhances public health by maximizing compliance of its regulated products and minimizing the risk associated with them
Health Resources and Services (HRSA) (51)	HRSA provides national leadership, program resources, and services needed to improve access to culturally competent, quality health care
Indian Health Service (IHS) (506)	Responsible for providing federal health services to American Indians and Alaska natives
National Institutes of Health (NIH) (110)	NIH is the nation's medical research agency, making important medical discoveries that improve health and save lives
Office of the Secretary (OS) (46)	The OS covers the mission of the DHHS, as well as the oversight for its more than 300 programs
Program Support Center (PSC) (21)	The PSC has a long tradition of providing support services to all components of the DHHS and other federal government agencies worldwide The PSC's broad range of more than 60 service and product offerings includes administrative operations, financial management, occupational health, human resources, and strategic acquisitions
Substance Abuse and Mental Health Services Administration (SAMSHA) (10)	The focus of SAMSHA is on building resilience and facilitating recovery for people at risk for mental or substance abuse disorders
US Marshals Service (USMS) (23)	The USMS is the enforcement arm of the federal courts, and as such, it is involved in virtually every federal law enforcement initiative. Nurses serve to promote prisoner health

To understand the role of Corps nurses, one must be familiar with the structure of the DHHS. They work in billeted positions that are related to the mission of the organization. For example, most nurses are assigned to the IHS (n = 506) and the BOP (n = 291). In the IHS, nurses work in clinical nursing jobs, providing care to members of the tribal organizations. In the BOP, most nurses are advanced practice nurses, and they provide primary care to the inmate populations.

How the Commissioned Corps Nurses Respond in Times of Need

Since 1798, the PHS has responded to domestic and global emergencies. Earlier, responses focused on epidemics and contagious diseases, such as smallpox, yellow fever, and cholera. At present, multidisciplinary teams respond to domestic and international humanitarian missions. Recent events include caring for Kosovo refugees as they arrived on US soil; workers at the site of the September 11 terrorist attacks in New York, New York (**Fig. 1**); and victims of the 2004 and 2005 tsunamis and earthquakes in Indonesia, as well as the 2005 hurricanes, Katrina and Rita.

How Deployments are Authorized Within DHHS

Different offices within the DHHS collaborate to provide assistance during disasters. Descriptions follow regarding 3 of the offices and their roles.

The Office of the Assistant Secretary for Preparedness and Response

Members of the Office of the Assistant Secretary for Preparedness and Response (ASPR) are the DHHS secretary's principal advisory staff for bioterrorism issues and other public health emergencies. ASPR coordinates interagency activities between DHHS, other federal departments, agencies, and offices and state and local officials

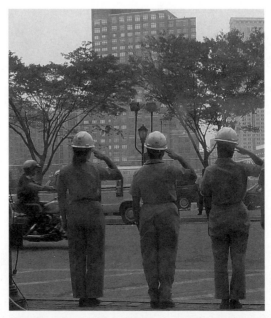

Fig. 1. A PHS nurse cares for a steel worker during the September 11 terrorist attacks in New York, New York (September 2001).

who are responsible for emergency preparedness and for protecting civilians from acts of bioterrorism and other public health emergencies.

The Offices of the Surgeon General and Public Health and Science

Within the Office of Public Health and Science is the OSG. It is within this office that the Commissioned Corps officers execute the emergency response component of their role in the PHS and the US government.

The Office of Force Readiness and Deployment

Housed in the OSG, the Office of Force Readiness and Deployment (OFRD) is responsible for training and deploying Corps officers during times of national and international public health need. OFRD has 3 major purposes:

- Build, monitor, and maintain the readiness capacity within the Corps;
- Ensure that officers are trained, protected, and ready to address urgent public health and medical needs; and
- Provide a rapid and effective response to domestic and international public health emergencies.

To ensure basic readiness to respond during times of national need, all Corps officers must meet readiness standards. To be qualified for deployment, minimum requirements must be met. The Corps officers must (1) have a current professional nursing license, (2) have a current Basic Life Support (BLS) certification, (3) have completed the Readiness Training Modules, (4) have received a current physical examination and medical history, (5) have received current immunizations, and (6) have passed the annual physical fitness test.

Nurses have a primary obligation to their assigned agency, but they also have responsibilities to the Corps. In addition to daily agency work, nurse officers are called to serve in temporary assignments. These may occur during war, such as backfilling as staff for deployed Department of Defense nurses at military treatment facilities, or in response to a national or public health emergency declared by the US president or the secretary of DHHS. Other occasions might include a response to an urgent public health need, such as critical staffing shortages causing a threat to the public health of a state, tribe, or local community, or a national security event declared by the secretary of Homeland Security.

COMMISSIONED CORPS RESPONSE TEAMS

The OFRD manages emergency response teams that are an essential part of the Corps and the PHS. Examples of such teams include a Rapid Deployment Force (RDF), an Applied Public Health Team (APHT), and an Incident Response Coordination Team.

The RDF provides mass casualty care that includes primary care, mental health, and public health services for a sheltered population. These teams may staff a Federal Medical Station (FMS) or a point-of-distribution operation where they provide mass prophylaxes and vaccinations. Other duties encompass providing medical surge capacity for local or state hospital or health facilities, isolation and quarantine prehospital triage, community outreach, and worldwide humanitarian assistance.

The APHT is composed of experts in public health assessments, environmental health, infrastructure integrity, food safety, vector control, epidemiology, and surveillance. The Incident Response Coordination Team performs liaison functions involving administration and finance logistics, communications, and planning.

Examples of services provided by the Commissioned Corps response teams during times of national and international need include

- Public health initiatives
  Immunizations;
  Food, water, and wastewater system assessments;
  Veterinary services; and
  Epidemiologic/public health consultation
- Direct medical care
  Primary/consultative care for children and adults;
  Dental care (eg, sealants, varnishes, restorations, and extractions); and
  Pharmacy support
- Infrastructure support
  Basic biomedical repair and training; and
  Environmental engineering
- Public health education
  Basic nursing skill training;
  Hand hygiene; and
  Basic life support, advanced cardiac life support, and pediatric advanced life support.

The OFRD designed a 4-tiered structure to deploy these teams. Teams in Tiers 1 and 2 include the RDF, the APHT, and the Mental Health Team (MHT). Tier 3 includes Corps officers who augment teams or mobilize as individual units when necessary. Tier 4 consists of Inactive Reserve and Medical Reserve Corps officers. **Table 2** depicts the tier structure and responsibilities within each tier.[5]

ROLE OF THE STRATEGIC NATIONAL STOCKPILE AND THE NATION'S FEDERAL MEDICAL STATIONS

Through DHHS, the Centers for Disease Control and Prevention (CDC) operate the Strategic National Stockpile (SNS). The SNS contains large quantities of medicine and medical supplies to protect the public when local supplies are depleted in case of a severe health emergency. Once federal and local authorities agree that the SNS is needed, medications and supplies can be delivered to any state within 12 hours. Each state is required to develop plans to receive and distribute the provisions to local communities as quickly as possible.

The CDC also maintains a cache of the FMSs, which are mobile units of medical supplies, equipment, and health care providers that provide medical care for evacuees with special needs. Each medical station has beds, supplies, and medicine to treat 250 people for a period determined by state and local needs without drawing resources from the host community.

As an integral part of emergency response, the FMSs provide surge capacity to undergird medical and public health systems that may be overwhelmed by mass casualties or displaced persons. The FMSs were originally intended to provide deployable medical capabilities (eg, equipment, materials, and pharmaceuticals) to assist hospitals in meeting surge requirements. Federal personnel staff the stations when deployed in support of regional, state, or local venues. Even when FMSs were in the early developmental stages, they were used in response to hurricanes Katrina and Rita. Ten 250-bed adaptations of the stations were created within days of Hurricane Katrina. Although the FMSs were designed to be staffed by federal personnel, they were adapted during the hurricanes to support state-run medical needs shelters. Current plans

Table 2			
Commissioned Corps response team structure			
Tier	**Team Characteristics and Responsibilities**		
Tiers 1 and 2	The RDF teams: • Report within 12 h • On call every 5 mo • 125 officers on the team (with specialists in clinical health, mental health, and applied public health)	The APHTs: • Report within 36 h • On call every 5 mo, with half the team serving as primary contacts • 47 officers on each team	The MHTs: • Report within 36 h • On call every 5 mo • 26 officers on each team
Tier 3	• Officers not assigned to Tier 1 or 2 teams • Have technical and subject matter expertise • Are "mission critical" employees—those designated by their agency to be nondeployable except in catastrophic circumstances		
Tier 4	Inactive Reserve Corps • Exists to provide surge capacity during times of acute need and to fill critical staffing shortages that may impair the service's ability to carry out the mission	Medical Reserve Corps • Exists to improve the health and safety of communities across the country by organizing and using public health, medical, and other volunteers	

are to expand the program to include stations that are specifically designed to support the states in providing care to evacuee populations with chronic medical conditions. As FMSs continue to develop, there is ongoing discussion regarding their use as quarantine stations in the event of a pandemic influenza epidemic.

COMMISSIONED CORPS NURSES DEFENDING THE PUBLIC HEALTH—ACTUAL DEPLOYMENTS

Since 1944, Commisioned Corps nurses have responded to domestic and international emergencies. **Table 3** shows examples of recent historic responses.

One of the largest PHS deployments to date occurred during 2005 in response to Hurricane Katrina in New Orleans, Louisiana. Hurricane Katrina was forecast to arrive on shore as a Category 5 storm. The Saffir-Simpson Hurricane Scale defines this type of hurricane as one with sustained winds greater than 155 mph.[6] Fortunately, it weakened to a strong Category 4 storm before making landfall, with sustained winds of 125 mph. The PHS teams were deployed from Washington, DC, and Atlanta, Georgia, the day before the storm hit.[7] An 800-bed field hospital was set up at the Pete Maravich Assembly Center, Louisiana State University in Baton Rouge, Louisiana, where the PHS nurses cared for more than 6000 patients during a period of 10 days. Hypertension and diabetes mellitus were the frequently diagnosed conditions. Nurses provided

Table 3 Examples of US PHS support missions	
PHS Missions	**Date**
Rwanda, Africa	1994
September 11 terrorist attacks, New York, New York	2001
Anthrax attacks, Washington, DC	2001
Fourth of July Celebration, National Capitol region, Washington, DC	2002
Tsumani, Southeast Asia	2002–2003
Winter Olympics, Salt Lake City, Utah	2002
Severe acute respiratory syndrome outbreak	2002–2003
Joint missions with the Department of Defense, Mercy Corps (a nongovernmental organization), current missions in South America	
Hurricane Katrina, Gulf States	2005
Hurricane Rita, Gulf States	2005
Hurricane Gustav, Texas and Gulf States	2008
2009 Presidential Inauguration, Washington, DC	2009
2009 State of the Union Address, Washington, DC	2009
H1N1 swine flu outbreak, Mexico and the world	2009

all levels of nursing care, from treating the most critical to the least critical, and caring for those with special needs.

The PHS also deployed Corps nurses to areas devastated by hurricanes Ike and Gustav in 2008.

One of the Corps nurses described the situation as follows:

"All of the PHS RDF teams deployed to hurricanes Ike and Gustav serving people in Louisiana, Texas, and Mississippi. RDF 1 set up and staffed the Federal Medical Station in College Station, Texas. At times the census of these high acuity patients was over 330. Team members, regardless of discipline, worked together to provide care to all evacuees. PHS nurses provided nursing care, including triage, physical assessment, medication administration, wound care, IV access and fluid administration, and activities of daily living. The patient population was diverse with many chronic medical problems, such as heart disease, hypertension, diabetes, renal disease, asthma, and chronic obstructive pulmonary disease (COPD). There were numerous individuals who were non-ambulatory, as well as those who were morbidly obese and unable to perform self care.

Nurses were scheduled for 12-hour shifts, providing around-the-clock care and monitoring for all evacuees, with many individuals working more than their scheduled shifts. Evacuees arrived at all times of the day or night. They came by the busload, private auto, as well as ambulance. Several busloads of people arrived within minutes of each other, which caused a tremendous surge of people seeking care.

Prior to the team's arrival, a complete 'hospital' was shipped from the Strategic National Stockpile. When the team arrived, it had all of the supplies, ie, beds, pharmacy, laboratory equipment, ventilators, to get the Federal Medical Hospital up and running. The medical station was restocked as necessary in accordance with the ability to get supplies to the station" (Braun Michelle, Hurricane Gustav Deployment, Personal Quotation, 2008).

Recently, the PHS nurses served as team members during the 2009 presidential inauguration in Washington, DC (**Fig. 2**). The PHS deployed 256 officers from all

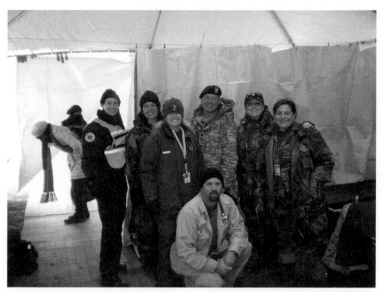

Fig. 2. The PHS nurses work side by side with Department of Defense and National Park Service personnel as they care for the 2009 presidential inauguration attendees.

disciplines to various locations, including the US Capitol grounds, along the National Mall, the headquarters of the DHHS, and assorted undisclosed locations. The primary on-site team was a PHS Tier 2 team, with additional staff assigned as needed. Approximately 100 members of this team were nurse officers who staffed first aid stations on the Mall or the US Capitol grounds. Others were assigned to medical stations in the DHHS building to distribute medication. In addition, the PHS nurses operated roaming BLS teams, walking in designated areas of the US Capitol and Mall. Teams were ready to provide needed care to thousands of people who attended the event. Given the diversity of the population, as well as the frigid weather conditions, the teams saw numerous cardiac, diabetic, hydration, and cold injuries. Approximately 750 patients were seen; Corps officers treated 697 of these patients, and 48% of the injuries were cold related.

The Corps also supports interservice, interagency health diplomacy initiatives as illustrated by its participation in Pacific Partnership 2009. This mission increased the operational capacity of US government personnel in delivering humanitarian assistance, which was given to developing countries and which focused on health promotion through performing public health assessments, conducting public health infrastructure repair, and providing training for indigenous health care workers.

In the past, the nurses were also part of the US Navy mission, Continuing Promise. During this humanitarian and civic assistance mission, Navy ships brought health care and other relief services to 8 Latin American and Caribbean nations. Humanitarian teams who served on the USS Kearsarge and USS Boxer provided medical care to 71,000 patients and conducted 348 surgeries and renovation projects. One of the participating nurses stated:

"During the fall of 2008, I was privileged to serve aboard the USS Kearsarge in support of Operation Continuing Promise 08. The USS Kearsarge was diverted from its original mission that was to the Dominican Republic. Instead, we helped with USAID relief efforts in Haiti after Hurricane Ike devastated the island. PHS officers performed health assessments; assessed water, supplies and sanitation; and immunized children. Other teams were flown to remote sites to provide primary medical care and immunizations to populations in the countries visited.

In October, we resumed our original mission with Continuing Promise and went to the Dominican Republic. There we worked side by side local military and civilian providers, nongovernment offices, partner military, and civilian professionals to provide medical, dental, optometry, and veterinary care at several sites throughout the island. During the 14-day operation, we conducted nearly 750 dental exams, 35 surgeries aboard the ship, and more than 2100 optometry exams. We also saw more than 16,000 patients for primary medical care and filled over 31,600 prescriptions." (Braun, USPHS)

In April 2009 United States faced an outbreak of swine flu (H1N1) virus. As a consequence of confirmed cases of swine influenza A (swH1N1) in California, Texas, Kansas, and New York, the acting secretary of the DHHS determined that a public health emergency existed nationwide and that the virus had significant potential to affect national security. This threat continues and is expected to remain at the forefront of the 2009 to 2010 influenza season. Corps nurses will respond as ordered by the Surgeon General to assist with efforts to contain and minimize the effects of such an epidemic.

SUMMARY

The Commissioned Corps of the PHS is one of 7 uniformed services whose mission is to protect, promote, and advance the health and safety of the United States. The PHS has a long history of delivering health promotion and disease prevention programs to all Americans and promoting the nation's public health. Corps nurses are the largest health profession represented in the PHS and are called on to deploy and respond with identified teams to national and international crises and disasters. Nurse officers serve in leadership positions in agencies of DHHS and the federal government and continue to standby to protect and defend the public health of the nation. Like individuals enlisted in sister military services with unique missions, the PHS nurse may serve "in harm's way" to protect and defend public health during times of need. Times of need are exemplified by past national emergencies, such as the terrorist and anthrax attacks of 2001, the 2004 to 2005 tsunamis and earthquakes in Indonesia, Hurricane Katrina, and the continuing threat of the H1N1 virus (swine flu). The PHS nurses demonstrate readiness through proper training. They are ready and willing to deploy in clinical and administrative roles to augment and support existing infrastructure and communities.

ACKNOWLEDGMENTS

The author wishes to extend special thanks to Lieutenant Commander Nichole J. Chamberlain, Senior Regulatory Science and Training Officer, Food and Drug Administration, Office of Regulatory Affairs, Division of Human Resource Development; Commander Kimberly Elenberg, Director, Training and Education, Office of Force Readiness and Deployment, Office of the Surgeon General; and Commander Patrick Denis, Deputy Director, Training and Education, Office of Force Readiness and Deployment, Office of the Surgeon General.

REFERENCES

1. US Department of Health and Human Services. About HHS. Availabe at: http://www.hhs.gov/about/.Published. Accessed July 25, 2009.

2. Mullan F. Plagues and politics. New York: Basic Books; 1989.
3. Parascandola JL. Public Health Service. In: Kurian GT, editor. A historical guide to the US government. New York: Oxford University Press; 1998. p. 487–93.
4. US Public Health Service Nursing. Chief nurse officer history. Available at: http://phs-nurse.org/chief-nurse/72-chief-nurse-history.html. Accessed July 25, 2009.
5. US Department of Health and Human Services. Commissioned corps response teams: a thumbnail sketch. Available at: http://ccrf.hhs.gov/ccrf/Response_Team_Description.htm.Published. Accessed July 26, 2009.
6. National Weather Service; National Hurricane Center. The Saffir-Simpson Hurricane Wind Scale (experimental). Available at: http://www.nhc.noaa.gov/aboutsshs.shtml.Published. Accessed August 16, 2009.
7. Debisette AT, Brown CR, Chamberlain N. A nursing perspective from United States Public Health Service nurses. J Prof Nurs 2006;22(5):270–2.

Ground Zero Recollections of US Public Health Service Nurses Deployed to New York City in September 2001

Ann R. Knebel, DNSc, RN[a,b,*], Angela M. Martinelli, PhD, RN, CNOR[a,c],
Susan Orsega, MSN, CRNP[a,d], Thomas L. Doss, RN, MPH[a,e],
Ana Marie Balingit-Wines, MPA, RN[a,f],
Carol L. Konchan, MSN, CRNP[a,g]

KEYWORDS

- US Public Health Service • Emergency preparedness
- September 11 • World Trade Center • Disaster response
- Public health service nursing

On September 11, 2001, now referred to as 9/11, the United States experienced a series of coordinated terrorist suicide attacks by air. Two passenger airplanes were hijacked by terrorists and flown into the World Trade Center (WTC) in New York City (NYC); a third plane was flown into the Pentagon in Northern Virginia; and a fourth plane crashed into the Pennsylvania countryside, after courageous

The views expressed in this manuscript do not necessarily represent the views of the US Department of Health and Human Services, the US Public Health Service, the Food and Drug Administration, the National Institutes of Health, the Department of Defense, or the United States Government.

[a] US Public Health Service Commissioned Corps (PHS CC), Office of Public Health and Science, US Department of Health and Human Services, 200 Independence Avenue SW, Washington, DC 20201, USA

[b] Office of the Assistant Secretary for Preparedness and Response, US Department of Health and Human Services, 200 Independence Avenue SW, Room 638 G, Washington, DC 20201, USA

[c] Division of Treatment and Recovery, National Institute on Alcohol Abuse and Alcoholism, 5635 Fisher Lane, Room 2028, Rockville, MD 20852, USA

[d] Division of Clinical Research/ Collaborative Clinical Research Branch, National Institute of Allergy and Infectious Disease, 6700 Rockledge Boulevard, Room 1122 Bethesda, MD 20892, USA

[e] Department of Defense TRICARE Management Activity, Skyline #5, Suite #810, 5111 Leesburg Pike, Falls Church, VA 22041, USA

[f] FDA Center for Devices and Radiological Health, US Department of Health and Human Services, Food and Drug Administration, Office of Compliance, Building 66, White Oak Campus, 10903 New Hampshire Avenue, Silver Spring, MD 20993, USA

[g] National Institute of Neurological Disorders and Stroke, US Department of Health and Human Services, National Institutes of Health, Building 10, Room 7C103, Bethesda, MD 20892, USA

* Corresponding author. Office of the Assistant Secretary for Preparedness and Response, US Department of Health and Human Services, 200 Independence Avenue SW, Room 638 G, Washington, DC 20201.
E-mail address: ann.knebel@hhs.gov

passengers thwarted a fourth attack that was likely targeted for the White House or US Capitol. These attacks tested the nation's response to public health and medical emergencies and stimulated unprecedented changes to the public health and medical response system, accelerating crucial transformations within the US Public Health Service Commissioned Corps (PHS CC) and in the way it responded to disasters and diseases.[1] In this article, the authors describe the roles and recollections of the nurses who deployed to "Ground Zero," the devastation area where the two WTC buildings once stood. The authors also briefly describe some of the changes that have now been instituted within the PHS CC in support of public health, medical, and human services responses to disasters.

BACKGROUND

The PHS originated, as decreed in legislation passed in 1798, "to provide for the accommodation of sick and disabled seamen" in hospitals at United States ports.[2] More than 70 years later, subsequent legislation created the position of supervising surgeon. The first supervising surgeon served in the Union Army during the Civil War and, recognizing the value of the military model of health care, required his physicians to wear military uniforms.[2] Over time, other professional categories were added to the uniform ranks, with nurses included in 1944.

From the beginning, the service comprised both commissioned officers and civilian personnel. During the 1960s, after an "avalanche of health-related legislation," the PHS was restructured and more leadership positions were given to civilian members of the service.[2] The PHS CC continued to uphold its mission of serving the public health of the nation, but the focus on the military model of uniformed service declined. In 1987, under the leadership of US Surgeon General C. Everett Koop, the uniformed Corps experienced a revitalization that included more frequent wearing of the uniform by CC officers and greater mobility in their assignments.[2] Revitalization continued under the leadership of subsequent US Surgeons General, who envisioned a broader role for PHS CC officers in responding to public health and medical emergencies.

The National Disaster Medical System (NDMS), was created in 1983 as a federally coordinated system to augment the nation's medical response capability.[3] The NDMS included Disaster Medical Assistance Teams (DMATs) to provide medical support. NDMS also includes veterinarian, and mortuary capabilities. These DMATs rapidly respond to help state and local authorities manage the medical impacts of major disasters. Most DMATs are composed of civilian personnel. One exception was the PHS-1 DMAT, which comprised PHS CC officers who served on the team as a volunteer duty. Despite its reliance on volunteers, the team maintained a defined structure, with field training opportunities and a cache of supplies.

Eleven years after the NDMS was established, the Commissioned Corps Readiness Force (CCRF) was created within the Office of the US Surgeon General to further augment national public health and medical response capabilities.[4] CCRF was initially just a list of names of PHS CC officers who agreed to be mobilized for deployments. When PHS CC officers are called to deploy to disaster locations, they must first be excused from their usual daily duties. Typically, PHS CC officers serve in various positions throughout the US Department of Health and Human Services (HHS), such as the US Food and Drug Administration and the National Institutes of Health, and in certain non-HHS federal agencies and programs, such as the Federal Bureau of Prisons.[5] These positions are in the areas of disease control and prevention; biomedical research; regulation of food, drugs, and medical devices; mental health and drug abuse; health care delivery; and international health.

In 1997, operational control of CCRF moved to the same office that managed the NDMS—the Office of Emergency Preparedness (OEP), located within the HHS, Office of the Assistant Secretary for Health.[4] Having experience with NDMS, OEP strengthened the CCRF by creating an operational database, establishing basic deployment requirements, and creating "ready-rosters" according to geographic location, home agency, and skills. This process helped ensure that the appropriate officers would be deployed, and prevented deploying too many officers from one region or agency simultaneously.

Before 9/11, PHS CC officers had deployed in support of various disaster-relief missions, such as the 1994 Northridge, California, earthquake to provide medical care; the 1999 Operation Provide Refuge at Fort Dix, New Jersey, to provide health assessments and immunizations for Kosovar refugees from the Balkan War; and the 2001 Tropical Storm Allison in Houston, Texas, to provide medical services to the local population and technical expertise regarding flood damage and mold remediation. The events of 9/11, however, set in motion the broadest emergency response ever conducted by the HHS,[6] and accelerated transformation of the Corps as people came to realize the tremendous potential of a uniformed service of 6000 public health and health care professionals.

The PHS CC nurses who authored this article deployed to NYC in the aftermath of that horrific day. Transformed by their experiences at Ground Zero, they have each contributed to the transformation of the Corps. This article shares those experiences and highlights the contributions and leadership of PHS CC nurses in public health and medical preparedness and response.

SITUATION REPORT

On September 11, 2001, at approximately 0845 hours Eastern Daylight Time, a commercial airplane crashed into the north tower of the WTC complex in NYC. At that time, the severity of the incident, the number of people involved, and the reason for the crash were all unknown. Shortly after 0900 hours, a second plane hit the WTC's south tower. At around 1000 hours, reports came in that another plane had hit the Pentagon in Northern Virginia, and a fourth plane was downed in Somerset County, Pennsylvania, about 80 miles southeast of Pittsburgh. Shortly after 1000 hours, the WTC's south tower collapsed, and within the next half-hour, the northern tower collapsed. (HHS Situation Report #1, 09/11/01, 2200 hours). Not long after the initial attack, a third building in the seven building WTC complex (**Fig. 1**) collapsed. This particular building housed the NYC Office of Emergency Management operations center. Consequently, the City's emergency response infrastructure had to be reestablished at an alternate location.

Many PHS CC officers were engaged immediately to support the response to these multiple events. By that evening, OEP had PHS CC officers in NYC and Shanksville, Pennsylvania, later OEP had PHS CC officers staffing the operations centers in three disaster locations—NYC, the Pentagon, and Somerset County, Pennsylvania (Rear Admiral Babb, personal communication, June 2009; at the time of the 9/11 response, Rear Admiral Babb was the director of the Commissioned Corps Readiness Force within the Office of the Assistant Secretary for Health and the director of emergency response operations for NDMS). Other officers supported the deployment of the Navy hospital ship, the USNS Comfort, both onboard the ship and through providing clinical "back fill" staffing at the National Naval Medical Center in Bethesda, Maryland, so that Naval personnel could deploy on the USNS Comfort to support the 9/11 response.

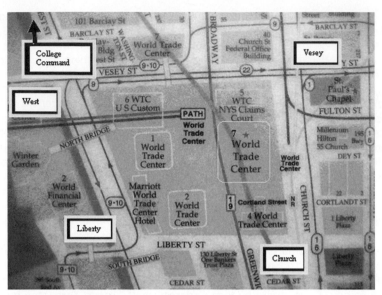

Fig. 1. Map of the World Trade Center Complex with the locations of first aid stations Vesey, West, Liberty, and Church. The College Command Post was located four blocks north of Barclay Street.

In the immediate aftermath of the attacks, local volunteers spontaneously set up ad hoc clinics in storefronts around Ground Zero. These unaffiliated volunteers had the best of intentions; however, without standardization or oversight, their rescue and relief services were neither regulated nor coordinated, and only contributed to the escalating chaos. On the night of September 12, NYC shut down all ad hoc operations and called in the NDMS supported the medical needs as part of an organized rescue and relief effort.

Five DMATs—one each from New York, New Jersey, and Rhode Island and two from Massachusetts—established medical operations around Ground Zero on September 14 (HHS Situation Report #1). During the following week, OEP began preparing to rotate in new DMATs to relieve the original five. One of the teams that rotated in was the PHS-1 DMAT, composed of volunteer-duty PHS CC officers; another team included 43 CCRF volunteer officers under the command of Captain (O-6) Kathleen Downs (Rear Admiral Babb, personal communication, June 2009).

The nurses who authored this article were part of the team that deployed under the command of Captain Downs. Participation in this deployment meant leaving their usual PHS CC jobs, which included supporting clinical and research programs for the National Institutes of Health (at the National Institute of Allergy and Infectious Diseases, the National Institute of Nursing Research, and the National Institute on Drug Abuse), supporting the Beneficiary Medical Programs for PHS CC personnel, and serving as a program analyst for the Vaccine Injury Compensation Program within the Health Resources and Services Administration.

DEPLOYMENT MISSION

On September 20, our team traveled by train to NYC. The mood on the train was somber; many of us were fearful of additional attacks, but having the opportunity to support the rescue efforts helped to minimize those fears. The team (**Fig. 2**) included both clinical providers (ie, physicians, nurse practitioners, physician assistants, nurses, pharmacists, and mental health practitioners) and nonclinical providers (ie, an engineer, an environmental health officer, physical therapists, and a health administrator), who assisted with logistics, communications, safety, and security.[7] For some team members, this was their first deployment.

When we arrived at Penn Station in NYC, it was disorienting with the cacophony of announcements, myriad of exits and trying to keep from losing any of our team in the crush of people. With the assistance of one of the team who knew the station we found the right exit where a bus was waiting to take us to the hotel. Arrangements had been made to have all response teams stay at a Sheraton Hotel in midtown Manhattan. Having seen the news with riveting details of the destruction, it felt strange to be staying at a hotel in Manhattan. The hotel staff welcomed us warmly; grateful for our assistance and also for the business because even though the train station had been busy the rest of the typically vibrant "Big Apple" was unusually quiet.

Our first rotation at Ground Zero was on the night shift. We traveled by bus with police escorts. Our first stop was at the College Command Post, set up at Manhattan Community College. There we were briefed about the mission and received our assignments, along with hard hats, goggles, and masks. We then walked to our assigned medical aid stations, which were set up on the perimeter of the rubble left by the towers, an area referred to as *the pile*, 16 acres of more than a million tons of debris (see **Fig. 1**). The bright lights illuminating the search and rescue work added to the surreal scene (**Fig. 3**).

To provide a sense of the magnitude of the destruction, a *New York Times* reporter wrote about the findings of a laser topographic mapping project of the surface of the disaster scene.[8] The data were given to firefighters and rescue workers to help them navigate the mounds and chasms of debris, and identify areas that could shift or collapse. All that was left of the 110 stories of WTC Towers 1 and 2 were two huge piles

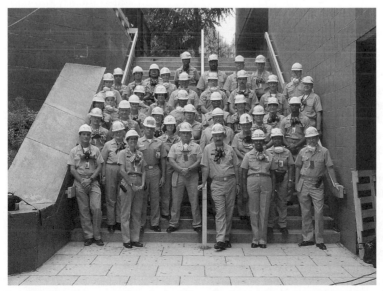

Fig. 2. The PHS CC–CCRF team that deployed to the World Trade Center on September 20, 2001.

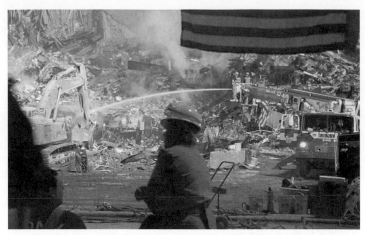

Fig. 3. The Church Street Aid Station at night. A mental health specialist talks with one of the rescue and recovery workers who visited the aid station.

of rubble, each one 60 ft high. The central plaza of the complex was a pit that sank 30 ft below street level. The Marriott WTC Hotel and WTC Building 7, which had housed the City's emergency operations center, were reduced to small mounds. Buildings 4 and 6 were partially collapsed and there was second 30-ft pit, Buildings 4 and 6 had partially collapsed. Rubble, fragments, and debris covered the roof of Building 5. Approximately 90,000 L of jet fuel had ignited the inferno that toppled the towers,[9] and fires continued to burn under the pile, significantly raising the surface temperature. Hot spots would flare as cranes lifted the wreckage. The intense fires continued to burn until October, and the last fire was not extinguished until December 20, 2001.[9]

When our team arrived 9 days after the attack, many of the responders on the scene obviously had gotten little sleep. They were still desperately searching to find anyone who might be alive in the pile. Smoke and dust permeated the air, and papers were strewn everywhere. A small cemetery behind the Vesey Street medical aid station was buried in papers several inches deep. Window blinds were wrapped around streetlights and tree branches. Years later, those indelible images remain with us, and we can still recall the smell of smoldering wreckage, acrid smoke, and burning plastic. We were reminded that this was a crime scene by the tight security and the posters telling people what to do if they found the black boxes from the airplanes that had brought down the towers.

Each passing day lessened the likelihood that anyone would be found alive, yet no one wanted to give up hope. The rescue workers and search dogs (**Fig. 4**) were visibly exhausted. One search dog handler said that the dogs were depressed because they were unable to recover any live victims. To raise their dogs' spirits, some of the handlers would hide in the debris so that the dogs could find them and think they had rescued victims. On September 26, 6 days after we arrived and 10 days after the last live victim was found, the mission switched from rescue to the recovery of remains.

During the deployment, our primary responsibility was to provide clinical care at the medical aid stations, not to participate in the actual rescue and recovery activities. When the mission switched from rescue to recovery, we began packing up unneeded equipment and supplies, because it was apparent that some of the first aid stations could be closed. We worked 8-hour shifts and rotated nights, days, evenings.

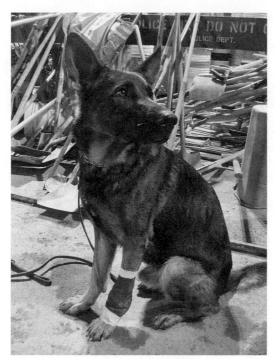

Fig. 4. The dogs that searched the pile worked tirelessly with their handlers seeking victims in the pile. Veterinarians were available (some through the NDMS) around the clock to tend to the needs of the search animals; note the bandage on the dog's leg. Booties were purchased to protect the pads of the dogs' feet from being injured by the heat from the fires and the sharp edges of the debris.

During our off time, we were encouraged to be "tourists" to help get things back to "normal." We did our laundry, watched the news, and read the papers, trying to make sense of the senseless act of terrorism. We called our families, kept journals, and tried to study. We took advantage of the restaurants, shows, and other activities NYC had to offer to help support the local economy that had been hard hit by the attack. Across the street from our hotel was the famous Carnegie Deli, which serves huge sandwiches named after theater and film stars. When we were on-duty, we would get wholesome, simple food from the Salvation Army or other charitable organizations that set up kitchens around the pile to serve the workers.

For those who were used to deploying to austere conditions (where you work long shifts, sleep on cots, have no running water, and electricity is provided by generators), this was an unusual deployment that created a bizarre sense of disconnection between the luxury of the hotel where we were staying and the complete desolation where we were working. But in typical NYC-style, luxury infiltrated the disaster scene when famous restaurants came to Ground Zero to provide gourmet meals for the workers, and stars, such as Susan Sarandon, helped serve the food.

PATIENTS TREATED IN THE AID STATIONS

The medical aid stations established by the DMATs began seeing patients on September 14, 3 days after the attack. Our team arrived on day 6 of the operations. Our patients were mostly firefighters, police personnel, and steel workers, many of whom were hesitant to enter the medical stations because they did not want to "waste time" when there were still people who needed to be saved. Our job was to make their clinic visits as quick as possible. Occasionally, if we were lucky, we could convince the patients to lie down to rest or accept a clean, dry pair of socks, and sometimes they would put their heads down and fall asleep immediately.

The medical stations remained open through November 19, 2001, although the number of stations declined over time. After the first 10 days, one station closed. Then, at weekly intervals, additional stations closed until there were only two medical aid stations operational for the last 6 weeks of the mission.

Perritt and colleagues[10] analyzed 9346 patient records from the five aid stations. Most of the patients were seen for "low-severity" complaints, such as minor trauma (eg, lacerations, burns, blisters), respiratory problems (eg, acute infections, rhinitis, obstructive pulmonary disease), eye complaints (eg, foreign bodies, irritation, traumatic injuries), headaches, digestive complaints (eg, reflux, gastritis), or skin problems (eg, dermatitis, infections). During the 10 weeks studied, only 171 of the complaints were categorized as moderate or high severity; these symptoms included chest pain, stroke, more severe respiratory and digestive problems, and traumatic injuries. Of these patients, 116 were transported to a hospital. The researchers also found that many of the visits to the medical aid stations could not be classified as an occupational injury or illness, but rather constituted requests for personal protective equipment and supplies, wellness/preventative checkups, counseling/support, or prescription refills.[10]

Although many injuries we treated were minor, the circumstances under which we provided care were within the context of a major disaster (**Fig. 5**). We tended to blisters, provided dry socks, washed out eyes, sutured lacerations, provided protective equipment, and gave people a place to rest and talk if they wanted. We were grateful for the opportunity to provide some comfort, especially as responders slowly realized that no one else would be found alive.

RECOLLECTIONS OF NURSES WHO DEPLOYED

The following vignettes are recollections of nurses who deployed to Ground Zero.

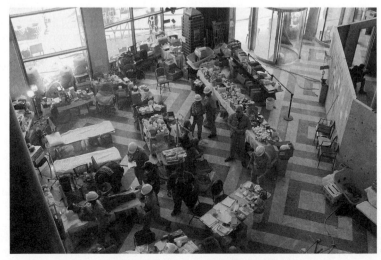

Fig. 5. The West Aid Station was set up in a damaged building.

Captain Angela Martinelli

I joined CCRF within months of transferring from the Army to PHS. Before 9/11, I had deployed to Fort Dix with Operation Provide Refuge to care for the victims of Yugoslavian ethnic cleansing and to Maniilaq Health Center in Kotzebue, Alaska, to assist in a nursing shortage.

On September 11, after finishing my duty day at the National Institute on Drug Abuse, I reported to the OEP and assisted with answering phones. Having served in the Army, I was accustomed to being on a Recall Roster, but at that time, PHS CC only had an informal recall process. When I left that day, I assured the director of the CCRF of my availability for whatever was needed. A few days later, the director phoned me, inquiring if I was available to go to Manhattan (Ground Zero). I remember my response was, "How could I not go!" Having grown up in Connecticut, NYC was home to me. However, this wasn't about my personal connection to NYC; it was about being a nurse on active duty and having an act of war occur on our soil. My duty was to be wherever there were people who needed care.

On the evening of September 20, the team gathered in a ballroom at the Sheraton Hotel in mid-Manhattan to receive a briefing. The individual who provided the briefing seemed to be completely disconnected from his surroundings. He had what is termed the *1000-yard-* or *2000-yard stare*. The latter phrase was popularized in 1945 when *LIFE Magazine* published the painting *That 2,000-Yard Stare* by World War II artist and correspondent Tom Lea.[11] The painting is a portrait of a young Marine at the Battle of Peleliu, which occurred in 1944. Call it battle fatigue, posttraumatic stress, or shell shock; whatever it is, it was all over the face of the man briefing us, and that of many others walking the halls of our hotel.

Our first shift began on Saturday, September 22, at midnight. As we gathered in the hotel lobby, I remember thinking how normal NYC looked in those surroundings, with its opulent shops and excessive prices. What was not normal, however, was that the lobby was not full of the usual visitors dressed to go to dinner or amble through Central Park in the fall. The lobby environment seemed more like a masquerade party, with people dressed in uniforms that each told their story: Central Intelligence Agency, Federal Bureau of Investigation, Federal Emergency Management Agency, and a host of fire, rescue, and police personnel from neighboring jurisdictions. I remember riding in an elevator with a Marine who looked at me in my uniform and said, "Remember, Commander [my uniform rank at the time], your mind is your primary weapon." I thought to myself, our primary weapon that can also be our primary enemy. I was only then imagining all the mental anguish and suffering that was to come.

One of the aid stations was positioned at Vesey Street, near the Millennium Hotel and next to a prayer station and the Salvation Army tent. Behind us was an old cemetery; I remember thinking, "the old dead looking on at the new." I peered into a coffee shop that was across the street. It was like a scene from the old television show *The Twilight Zone*. Time had stopped. There were racks full of donuts and coffee cups were still on the counter, but the interior was filled with rubble, dust, and debris. The clock on the wall had stopped. The entire Ground Zero was like a Hollywood set. It was surreal.

Our mission was basic nursing care Florence Nightingale style. Drink water, have something to eat, have a pair of clean socks. I thought of Nightingale's *Notes on Nursing,* which describes nursing as "the proper use of fresh air, light, warmth, cleanliness, quiet, and proper selection and administration of diet—all at the least expense of vital power to the patient."[12] For the next 10 days, that was our job—to nurse the sick. But for the most part, all we could offer was a hand of comfort, a listening ear, and a compassionate look.

These simple, small gestures are really the essence of nursing: to care for the wounded not only physically but also spiritually and emotionally as they face the demons of fear, anger, pain, and grief, and the uncertainty of what is to come.

Captain Susan Orsega

I remember vividly the moments when we were slowly approaching the scene of the destruction for the first time. It was nighttime; my senses were overwhelmed. As the bus drove down the streets, we could hear loud cheers from onlookers who were awake late at night to support us. We were given badges and masks, and were quickly shuffled through security and incoming briefs. I'll never forget my initial reaction when hearing the huge cranes screeching as they picked up large fractured pieces of the buildings. The sound was so piercing it was as if the buildings were crying from all the lost lives. I thought: "I can do this."

I think my words included in the *NIH Record* sum up the thoughts of many who experienced Ground Zero. Despite witnessing indescribable horror, I felt "honored [to be] responding on behalf of the nation. There were so many good people that were there. The fire fighters were never, ever going to stop...so many people lost their friends. It was a war zone, really."[13] Responding as a nurse practitioner, I examined patients who had muscular skeletal overuse injuries, respiratory illnesses, and ocular injuries. It felt like these examinations were windows to the soul; I would often end my examinations by asking the patient about their mental health. Sometimes patients would not really have a specific complaint but wanted to come into the tent for respite from their physical and mental exhaustion. The mental health providers assigned to the team had an instrumental role.

Captain Tom Doss

What I took from the event was the self-sacrifice and resiliency of the local population. I had the sense that many of them would take emotional scars with them. The fragility of human life became evident, and maybe for this reason the remains of those who died were treated with the utmost respect. One vivid memory was the line of ambulances waiting for remains. When remains were found, everything stopped. The remains were gently put on a litter and covered with an American flag. They were then put into an ambulance and slowly driven away with lights flashing.

Captain Carol Konchan

Like Captain Martinelli, I joined CCRF early and deployed in support of Operation Provide Refuge. I remember feeling a sense of pride at being asked to deploy to NYC. I had watched the news coverage of the attacks on the WTC and the Pentagon and had worried that there would be more attacks in the Washington, DC, area, where I worked for the Health Resources and Services Administration. Little did I know that my own family members, who lived in southwestern Pennsylvania, saw and heard the Flight 93 plane before it crashed near Shanksville. Deploying to Ground Zero gave me a personal link to each of the sites attacked that day.

Walking to the first aid stations that first night, I was transfixed by the magnitude and enormity of the damage—it was so extensive, it was hard for me to take it all in. So many buildings were gone. The buildings still standing had massive damage. One building looked as if a monstrous cat had taken its huge paw and scratched away the exterior, revealing the offices, with the desks and chairs still there. I felt like I *knew* the victims personally. Displayed everywhere were posters, photographs, names of victims, and small memorials. There was a sense of unity in the initial days after 9/11. Teams came from everywhere. Everyone wanted to do something to help. The workers just refused to quit. It was not unusual to see a worker sitting on the sidewalk, propped up against a building, sound asleep.

It was a great honor to have been selected to represent the PHS CC and work alongside the DMAT teams. It was reassuring to work with team members I knew and to build new friendships with those I did not. The support and sense of patriotism displayed in the aftermath of the 9/11 attacks will be memories that will stay with me forever.

Captain Ana Marie Balingit-Wines

I served as the chief nurse for the deployment to Ground Zero. This deployment was extremely painful and traumatic for me. I spent considerable time during college in that area of Manhattan. Seeing the devastation and familiar landmarks gone—no, decimated—was more than I could handle. Remembering the feeling I had that first time we set foot on Ground Zero still brings tears to my eyes. Perhaps it's remembering the stoicism and pain of the tough firefighters and police officers working on the pile, or the helplessness I felt in attempting to console them whenever they came in for medical treatment that makes me sad.

In retrospect, having served for 5 years as the chief nurse for NDMS, my takeaway message would be the importance of cooperation and working collaboratively across all agencies involved in disaster response. For example, I recall how difficult it was to travel between the hotel and Ground Zero without police escort. Having the police cooperate with the people who were coordinating our transportation allowed the medical teams to travel more quickly to the disaster scene. The lessons learned from responding to events such as 9/11 and Hurricane Katrina, and the continuous dialog between the agencies involved have significantly improved national preparedness and response operations.

LESSONS LEARNED

The deployment to the WTC was successful in many respects. The care given at the aid stations provided workers who searched the pile and removed the debris not only essential occupational health services but also personal protective equipment, supplies, counseling, and support. The PHS CC nurses played a unique role in this mission, providing care and comfort to the workers, many of whom had the "1000-yard stare" and who were slowly coming to grips with the fact that many of their friends and colleagues had perished. The nurses who deployed showed leadership by helping bring order and calm to the chaos. They provided a holistic approach to caring for the patients, giving those they encountered the courage to endure and hope for the future.

Beyond the immediate care provided, the deployment also accelerated the transformation of the PHS CC back to its roots as a uniformed service. Officers now wear uniforms daily, a deployment team structure has been implemented, and all officers must meet deployment standards. In 2001, most training was completed "online" and not required. Now, educational preparedness is required for every PHS CC officer, and includes classroom, online, and field training, with nurses at the forefront of developing these educational programs. The missions have become increasingly frequent, and nurses are critical components of any deployable medical team, not only as clinicians but also as part of the team's leadership.

Combined missions with other response teams have also become more common. The WTC deployment of PHS CC officers was the beginning of combined DMAT–PHS CC missions. As mentioned in the article by Debisette and colleagues in this issue, collaboration and melding of expertise has become the standard for National Special Security Events, such as staffing the first aid stations during the annual 4th of July celebration in Washington, DC.

Joint missions with the Department of Defense are also more common. For example, PHS CC officers continue to support Department of Defense humanitarian missions, such as Pacific Partnership 2009 and Continuing Promise 2009. Pacific Partnership 2009 provides humanitarian civic assistance and teams of preventive medicine, veterinarian, medical, and dental personnel in the Asia-Pacific region. Continuing Promise 2009 shows US commitment and support to Latin America and the Caribbean region through providing medical services and humanitarian assistance.

For the WTC mission, some of the deploying personnel had participated in previous deployments or had prior military service; for others, the deployment to Ground Zero was their first field experience. Officers now participate in exercises that simulate austere field conditions to prepare personnel for work in that type of environment. Deployment roles are better defined, and more rigorous clinical training and physical fitness requirements have been instituted.

Worker safety was a particular concern during the WTC response. Toxic fires were not completely extinguished until December 2001. Content of the toxic fumes was not tested in the first 24 hours, when the plume was most intense; thousands of trained responders and unaffiliated volunteers converged at the WTC site before protective equipment was readily available to everyone. Because of the emotionally charged atmosphere and confusion over boundaries of authority—key leaders were lost in the building collapses and the emergency operations center was destroyed—site management and perimeter control were initially chaotic.[9] The medical aid stations provided masks and conducted fit testing (**Fig. 6**) according to the strong recommendations of the National Institute for Occupational Safety and Health; but for the most part, people did not wear their masks[14] and were exposed to toxic substances for prolonged periods.

During the course of the site clean-up, which officially ended in May 2002, the settled dust was tested and found to contain an alkaline mixture of construction materials that can be particularly corrosive to the respiratory tract.[15] In 2002, the WTC Worker and Volunteer Medical Screening Program was established to characterize

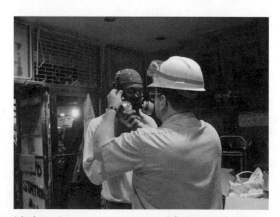

Fig. 6. Officers provided respiratory protection and fit testing for the workers who came to the clinic without equipment.

WTC-related health effects.[16] The program provided free standardized examinations to responders between July 2002 and April 2004. In 2006, results of the medical screening program reported that 69% of 9442 responders experienced new or worsened respiratory symptoms, with persistence in 59% of these workers.[16]

In addition to the pulmonary complications for those who responded, mental health concerns remain a large issue. The WTC Health Registry is a voluntary registry of people who were exposed to the terrorist attack, and includes nearly 30,000 rescue/recovery workers.[17] From these WTC Health Registry data, Perrin and colleagues[17] reported that the overall prevalence of posttraumatic stress disorder among 28,962 workers was 12.4%, with the highest prevalence (21.2%) in unaffiliated volunteers, such as the health care providers that spontaneously deployed to the disaster scene to help. Other psychiatric morbidities also have been reported and include depression and panic disorder as the most prevalent.[18]

WHAT HAS CHANGED

The responses to 9/11, the anthrax attacks, and Hurricane Katrina have stimulated sweeping changes regarding how the federal government responds to disasters.[19] Legislation created the Department of Homeland Security. Numerous presidential directives have been issued that address national preparedness and response. For example, the Federal Response Plan is now the National Response Framework (NRF), and emphasizes integration of preparedness and response starting locally and expanding if federal support is needed. The National Incident Management System was created to standardize the approach to incident management to include Incident Command System principles.

To address the environmental safety lessons from the WTC response, a worker safety annex was added to the NRF. The Occupational Safety and Health Administration coordinates federal assets for worker safety and health, which is an important step forward but only pertains to federal responders. An integrated and scalable multiagency safety management function must be built into the incident command system to protect the entire response workforce.[9]

Ensuring that responders are "fit for duty," both physically and emotionally, has also become a crucial element for personnel performing response activities. On January 1, 2002, the definition and training requirements of a "deployable" officer in the PHS CC were made policy.[20] Subsequently, CCRF was subsumed into the Office of Force Readiness and Deployment, within the office of the US Surgeon General, to further strengthen the deployment readiness of the PHS CC.[21]

In June 2002, Congress passed legislation that established the Office of Public Health Emergency Preparedness within HHS. This office was charged with performing activities to prepare for and respond effectively to bioterrorism and other public health emergencies. In the subsequent Pandemic and All Hazards Preparedness Act passed in December 2006, the Office of Public Health Emergency Preparedness became part of the Office of the Assistant Secretary for Preparedness and Response (ASPR). The legislation consolidated the responsibilities for federal public health and medical emergency preparedness and response within the ASPR office.

ASPR has the responsibility of coordinating the federal public health and medical response to disasters as directed under the Emergency Support Function #8 Annex of the NRF. ASPR works with its support agencies (eg, Department of Defense, Department of Veterans Affairs) and the PHS CC to assure robust public health and medical support to states during disasters. PHS CC nurses not only provide public health, mental health, and clinical care to disaster victims but also serve in leadership roles. For example, nurses provide leadership for the HHS headquarters Emergency Management Group, which executes the federal public health and medical response in support of states' requests for assistance. Likewise, nurses lead the Incident Response Coordination Team, which coordinates the integration of federal assets into the local response.

Within ASPR, the Office of Preparedness Planning leads the development of playbooks that define how ASPR will coordinate the federal public health and medical response to specific scenarios. This office also has regional emergency coordinators stationed throughout the country. These emergency coordinators engage state/local preparedness agencies to analyze gaps, anticipate response missions, and assist in proactively deploying assets to meet states' requests for assistance. Each response is analyzed to determine the lessons observed so that corrective actions can be taken to address issues and constantly improve preparedness and response operations. Again, PHS CC nurses are at the forefront of many of these preparedness and response activities. **Table 1** provides references to Web sites for additional information on each of these advances in how the federal government responds to disasters.

As shown by the missions that PHS CC nurses have supported before and since the WTC disaster, this cadre of nursing professionals is leading preparedness efforts and stands ready to respond at a moment's notice to rapidly and effectively deliver federal assistance in support of the public health, medical, and human services needs of the nation. The reflections of the authors of this article mirror the commitment of the entire nurse Corps of the US PHS to this mission.

Table 1	
Milestones and Web site references to federal disaster preparedness and response	
Milestones	**Web Site**
Created the Department of Homeland Security	http://www.dhs.gov/index.shtm
Issued numerous Presidential Directives	http://www.fas.org/irp/offdocs/nspd/index.html
The Federal Response Plan become the National Response Framework	http://www.fema.gov/emergency/nrf/
Created a Worker Safety Annex to the National Response Framework	http://www.fema.gov/pdf/emergency/nrf/nrf-support-wsh.pdf
Created the National Incident Management System	http://www.fema.gov/emergency/nims
Established PHS CC Office of Force Readiness and Deployment	http://ccrf.hhs.gov/ccrf/
Created the Office of Public Health Emergency Preparedness within the Department of Health and Human Services	http://www.upmc-biosecurity.org/Website/resources/govt_legislation/crs_summaries/public_health_sec_act_crs_summary.html
Created the Office of the Assistant Secretary for Preparedness and Response	http://www.hhs.gov/aspr
Updated Emergency Support Function #8 annex (public health and medical services) within the National Response Framework	http://www.fema.gov/pdf/emergency/nrf/nrf-esf-08.pdf
Developed playbooks for responding to pubic health and medical emergencies	http://www.hhs.gov/disasters/discussion/planners/playbook/

Abbreviation: PHS CC, Public Health Service Commissioned Corps.

POSTSCRIPT

The nurses who served at Ground Zero continue to serve as leaders in support of national public health and medical preparedness and response. Captain Martinelli served as a deployment coordinator for Office of Force Readiness and Deployment for more than 4 years and regularly deploys. Captain Orsega has deployed more than 10 times and has supported several Department of Defense–sponsored humanitarian missions. Captain Doss served as the administration and finance officer for the ASPR emergency management group that executes the federal public health and medical response. Captain Konchan returned from Ground Zero and several days later reported to the National Naval Medical Center to augment staffing. She has supported many other deployments. Captain Balingit-Wines served for 5 years as the chief nurse of the NDMS, which augments the national medical response capability. Rear Admiral Knebel returned to NYC in September 2002 for 9 months to assist the Office of Emergency Management with bioterrorism planning efforts. Currently, as deputy director for preparedness planning in ASPR, she is responsible for developing the plans to coordinate the federal public health and medical response.

REFERENCES

1. PHS CC transformation information page. U.S. Public Health Service Commissioned Corps Web site, 2009. Available at: http://usphs.gov/transformation. Accessed July 6, 2009.
2. Mullan F. Plagues and politics: the story of the United States Public Health Service. New York: Basic Books; 1989.
3. Knouss RF. National disaster medical system. Public Health Rep 2001; 116(Suppl 2):49–52.
4. OFRD history. Office of Force Readiness and Deployment Web site, 2009. Available at: http://ccrf.hhs.gov/ccrf/ccrf_essentials.htm. Accessed July 6, 2009.
5. About the PHS CC agencies page. U.S. Public Health Service Web site, 2008. Available at: http://www.usphs.gov/aboutus/agencies.aspx. Accessed July 6, 2009.
6. Babb J, Beck D. The U.S. Public Health Service providing care and leadership. The Officer 2001;77(10):15–7.
7. Downs K, Balingit-Wines AM. CCRF members deployed to WTC. Commissioned Corps Bulletin 2001;15(11):5–8.
8. Chang K. From 5,000 feet up, mapping terrain for Ground Zero workers, vol. 150. New York Times. September 23, 2001; Section B1:1.
9. Reissman DB, Howard J. Responder safety and health: preparing for future disasters. Mt Sinai J Med 2008;75(2):135–41.
10. Perritt KR, Boal WL. The Helix Group. Injuries and illnesses treated at the World Trade Center, 14 September–20 November 2001. Prehosp Disaster Med 2005; 20(3):177–83.
11. Lea T. Marines call it that 2,000-yard stare: paintings from the Battle of Peleliu. Life 1945;18(24):65.
12. Nightingale F. Notes on nursing: what it is, and what it is not. London: Harrison & Sons; 1859. p. 8.
13. McManus R. At Ground Zero: NIH'ers respond to tragedy in NYC. NIH Record, October 30, 2001. Available at: http://nihrecord.od.nih.gov/newsletters/10_30_2001/main.htm. Accessed July 6, 2009.

14. Feldman DM, Baron SL, Bernard BP, et al. Symptoms, respirator use, and pulmonary function changes among New York City firefighters responding to the World Trade Center disaster. Chest 2004;125(4):1256–64.
15. Lioy PJ, Weisel CP, Millette JR, et al. Characterization of the dust/smoke aerosol that settled east of the World Trade Center (WTC) in lower Manhattan after the collapse of the WTC 11 September 2001. Environ Health Perspect 2002;110(7): 703–14.
16. Herbert R, Moline J, Skloot G, et al. The World Trade Center disaster and the health of the workers: five-year assessment of a unique medical screening program. Environ Health Perspect 2006;114(12):1853–8.
17. Perrin MA, DiGrande L, Wheeler K, et al. Differences in PTSD prevalence and associated risk factors among World Trade Center disaster rescue and recovery workers. Am J Psychiatry 2007;164(9):1385–94.
18. Stellman JM, Smith RP, Katz CL, et al. Enduring mental health morbidity and social function impairment in World Trade Center rescue, recovery, and cleanup workers: the psychological dimension of an environmental health disaster. Environ Health Perspect 2008;116(9):1248–53.
19. Sauer LM, McCarthy ML, Knebel AR, et al. Major influences on hospital emergency management and disaster preparedness. Disaster Med Public Health Prep 2009;3(Suppl 2):S68–73.
20. Babb J. Changes in the CCRF operations plan. Commissioned Corps Bulletin, January 5–6, 2002. Available at: http://dcp.psc.gov/ccBulletin/PDF_docs/Jan02ccb.pdf. Accessed July 6, 2009.
21. Federal Register Notice dated December 18, 2003. Vol. 68, No. 243. Available at: http://edocket.access.gpo.gov/2003/03-31242.htm. Accessed July 6, 2009.

Development of an Evidence-Based Pressure Ulcer Program at the National Naval Medical Center: Nurses' Role in Risk Factor Assessment, Prevention, and Intervention Among Young Service Members Returning from OIF/OEF

David R. Crumbley, MSN, RN, Michele A. Kane, PhD, RN*

KEYWORDS

- Evidence-based nursing care • Military • Pressure ulcers
- Pressure ulcer development • Wound care

Because the terms *decubitus ulcer* and *bed sore* leave many people believing these wounds are the result of lying in bed, they have been replaced with the term *pressure ulcer*. According to the National Pressure Ulcer Advisory Panel, "pressure ulcer is localized injury to the skin and/or underlying tissue usually over a bony prominence, as a result of pressure, or pressure in combination with shear."[1] The war wounded are not immune to pressure ulcer development and unfortunately, as a result of the severity of their injuries and the process of medical evacuation, the risk for pressure

The opinions or assertions contained herein are solely the views of the authors and should not be construed as official or reflecting the views of the Department of Defense or United States Government.
Copyright statement: The authors were employees of the U.S. Federal Government when this work was conducted and prepared for publication. Therefore, it is not subject to the Copyright Act, and copyright cannot be transferred.

National Naval Medical Center, 8901 Wisconsin Avenue, Bethesda, MD 20889-5600, USA
* Corresponding author.
E-mail address: michele.kane@med.navy.mil

Nurs Clin N Am 45 (2010) 153–168
doi:10.1016/j.cnur.2010.02.009
0029-6465/10/$ – see front matter. Published by Elsevier Inc.

nursing.theclinics.com

ulcer development in the young wounded returning from Iraq and Afghanistan has increased. Furthermore, the risk for pressure ulcers has been actualized, with one of the major military treatment centers noting an increase in the incidence of pressure ulcers among the returning wounded.

The use of military munitions or improvised explosive devices (IEDs) results in signature wounds and severe battlefield injuries. The unique nature of the materials used in these weapons and the severity of injuries caused by them increases the risk for polytrauma-related complications, including pressure ulcers. The incidence of pressure ulcers has increased in casualties returning from Operation Iraqi Freedom (OIF) and Operation Enduring Freedom (OEF) from 2003 to the present. One current widely accepted tool for assessing risk for pressure ulcer development is the Braden scale. However, protocols using some assessment tools may be limited, because few nursing interventions correspond to the risk level identified by the assessment tool.

BACKGROUND

Discussions of pressure ulcers among the military wounded go back as early as the 16th century when Ambrose Pare, one of the founding fathers of surgery, spoke of the management of pressure ulcers in a wounded French aristocrat.[2] However, the phenomenon of pressure ulcer development among military service members and casualties was not an issue during World War I and conflicts before that period. Most casualties who experienced severe spinal cord injuries during those previous conflicts and wars unfortunately did not survive their initial injuries.

Attention to this phenomenon began to change in the 1940s when Donald Munro[3] wrote about the dramatic increase in the incidence of pressure ulcers among the war wounded during World War II. At Cushing Veterans' Administration General Hospital from 1946 to 1947, the percentage of patients who developed a pressure ulcer before discharge was as high as 69%. During this same period, the incidence of pressure ulcers in civilian facilities was 28%.[3] In World War II, plaster of Paris jackets were the only available method for stabilizing the spine of patients who had spinal cord injuries during transport. Unfortunately, this practice produced significantly high skin/cast interface pressures, and repositioning the patient was not effective in reducing pressure.

Since the Global War on Terror began in 2001, the patient population within military treatment facilities (MTFs) has changed significantly. Before the Global War on Terror, MTFs treated patients a mix of typical medical and surgical conditions, with a limited number of trauma patients. The trauma patients were usually those who had injuries acquired in motor vehicle crashes or military training accidents. Currently, the patient population in MTFs, particularly the larger teaching hospitals, consists of a greater number of young patients who have polytrauma and were injured by explosions secondary to IEDs.

IEDs contain extreme explosive force capable of permanently disabling a tank or other armored vehicle. Therefore, these blasts have a devastating effect on the human body, resulting in amputations, fractures, large soft-tissue defects, brain and spinal cord injuries, and even death.

Immediate resuscitative care for people with these injuries often occurs in an austere environment and at the onset focuses on the life-saving interventions of advanced trauma life support. As soon as the injured individuals are medically stabilized in a hospital in the war zone, a military medical aircraft transports them to Landstuhl Regional Medical Center (LRMC), Germany. Once there, they undergo further surgical interventions and stabilization for their trip back to the United States. From

LRMC, they are transported to one of two major MTFs: Walter Reed Army Medical Center (WRAMC) in Washington, DC, or the National Naval Medical Center (NNMC) in Bethesda, Maryland. Both facilities are on the East Coast and within 10 miles of each another. Patients who have severe burns are transported to Brook Army Medical Center (BAMC) in San Antonio, Texas, where the United States Institute of Surgical Research, also known as the Army's Burn Center, is located.

UNUSUALLY SUSCEPTIBLE POPULATIONS

Before the Global War on Terror, MTFs did not commonly have an elevated prevalence or incidence of pressure ulcers in the younger age group represented by the current patient population in the larger military medical centers. Although young and healthy before their injury, these patients are typically dealing with spinal cord injuries, traumatic brain injury, multiple amputations, or large soft tissue injuries. Pressure ulcers are characteristically more prevalent in individuals aged 18 to 30 years because of spinal cord injuries and in those older than 65 years because of advancing age and failing health.[4] As shown in **Fig. 1**, this new population of young polytrauma patients has created new challenges for the military health care system, one of which is preventing pressure ulcer development. The injuries were most likely sustained in a hostile and austere environment where care is focused primarily on immediate life-threatening interventions and on medical evacuation to a higher level of care. Medical evacuation most likely will occur on a NATO field litter, which can produce peak interface pressures greater than 30 mm Hg over bony prominences.[5] The combination of polytrauma, traumatic brain injury, hypoperfusion, sedation, cervical collars, and medical evacuation places injured individuals at high risk for pressure ulcer development early in the care continuum.

SIGNIFICANCE

In 2007, health care providers at the bedside at NNMC perceived an increase in the incidence of pressure ulcer development in its young service members. The returning casualties from OIF and OEF apparently had a significantly increased risk for developing pressure ulcers. A review of NNMC patient data from 2003 to 2007 verified an increasing frequency of young patients developing a pressure ulcer during hospitalization (**Figs. 1** and **2**). These pressure ulcer incidences included patients who had

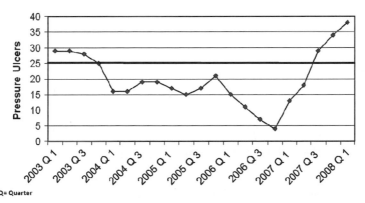

Q= Quarter

Fig. 1. National Naval Medical Center pressure ulcers per 1000 discharges 2003–2008: stay longer than 4 days.

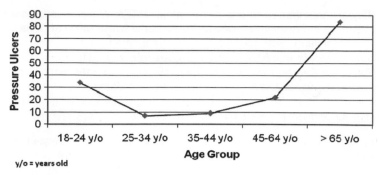

Fig. 2. National Naval Medical Center pressure ulcer incidence by age group: 2005–2007.

a hospital stay of 4 days or longer, and the rate was risk-adjusted per 1000 discharges. The rate increased from 16 incidences per 1000 discharges in the first quarter of 2007, to 34 incidences per 1000 discharges by the fourth quarter of 2007.

NNMC uses the Agency for Health care Research and Quality (AHRQ) 2009 national hospital benchmark for pressure ulcers, which is 25.1 incidences per 1000 discharges overall and 5.22 incidences per 1000 discharges in the 18-to 39-year-old age group. The increase in pressure ulcers seen in the NNMC patient population greatly exceeded this standard.[6]

The increase in pressure ulcer occurrence was concerning, but even more concerning was the rise in pressure ulcer incidence among the 18- to 25-year-old patients who had been wounded in combat (see **Fig. 1**). These patients were developing pressure ulcers to the occipital region, sacrum, heels, and various locations on the feet at a more frequent rate than had been observed previously. In some cases, the pressure ulcers were severe enough to require surgical intervention with plastic surgery.

DEVELOPMENT OF AN EVIDENCE-BASED PRESSURE ULCER PREVENTION PROGRAM

In an effort to correct this problem, an evidence-based practice (EBP) project for pressure ulcer prevention was initiated in early 2008 at NNMC. During the initial phase of the EBP project, the current NNMC pressure ulcer process manual was thoroughly reviewed to gain an understanding of which nursing practices were not being effectively used.

Inclusion and Exclusion Criteria

Articles identified by searches of the PubMed, CINAHL, and Ovid databases were reviewed at the start of the EBP project. Search terms included bedsores, war wounded, combat wounded, pressure ulcer management, pressure ulcer guidelines, head injury, and spinal cord injury. Inclusion criteria included all study types. Most literature reviewed had been published within the past 10 years, but some articles before 1995 were included for basic medical reference and historic perspective. Studies not written in English were excluded.

REVIEW OF LITERATURE RELATED TO PRESSURE ULCERS

Historically, studies related to military veterans have focused on pressure ulcers in the noncombatant Veterans Administration (VA) rehabilitation settings. The review of the literature showed that limited research has addressed young combatant patients directly from the battlefield. In a review of the literature from 2000 to 2009, the authors located 2450 references pertaining to pressure ulcers. In addition to the journal articles, multiple clinical guidelines and toolkits for pressure ulcer prevention are available. Selection of guidelines and toolkits for review was based on examination of the most current research on pressure ulcer prevention and management. One guideline, developed by the Institute for Healthcare Improvement (IHI) as part of the "Protecting 5 Million Lives from Harm" campaign, was used throughout this EBP project.[7]

The literature review found limited studies discussing pressure ulcers and specifically examining the combat wounded during hospitalization at an MTF. Much of the literature discussing pressure ulcers in military veterans focused on patients within the VA health care system who had spinal cord injury. These studies were not specific to the combat wounded; they included multiple origins and environments. An exception was a study discussing pressure ulcers among military veterans returning from OIF or OEF; it focused on wounded within a VA facility who had been treated and later discharged from an MTF.[8]

The relationship between MTFs and VA facilities is important with respect to service members' health care for three reasons. First, MTFs are the treatment centers in the federal health care system, whereas the VA centers are the facilities that render rehabilitation care. A large number of injured service members require years of rehabilitation. Second, not all service members (guard or reserve) live near large MTFs such as NNMC or WRAMC, and therefore the VA centers are located throughout the United States to provide rehabilitative care to injuries sustained from OIF and OEF. Third, after completion of military service, honorably discharged service members, who are then considered veterans, can receive health care from any VA facility within the United States. This important continuation of health care is built into the U.S. National Federal system. Without the collaboration between the MTFs and VA centers to provide care for service members, a large number of injured veterans would not be able to return home and seek further care, and would need to reside closer to larger MTFs in the United States.

Through a retrospective chart review, Harrow and colleagues[8] found that the risk for a service member arriving at a VA polytrauma rehabilitation center (PRC) in Tampa, Florida, with a pressure ulcer was 53% for those wounded in Iraq compared with 22% for service members wounded in an area other than Iraq. This finding is significant because it indicates the existence of a pressure ulcer problem before patients were admitted into a VA health care facility, and suggests that the ulcer occurred somewhere in the continuum of care before the patient entered the VA health care system.

IDENTIFIED ISSUES AND PROBLEMS ASSOCIATED WITH THE POTENTIAL FOR PRESSURE ULCERS IN YOUNG MILITARY SERVICE MEMBERS

As the authors further developed the evidence-based pressure ulcer program, they identified some significant issues and problems related to the younger military population, pressure ulcer development, and the lack of significant literature. For example, none of the reviewed research studies address the long-term effects of pressure ulcers in a younger military population. Likewise, none of the reviewed studies related to pressure ulcers discuss whether specific treatments or nursing interventions have a direct correlation to the prevention of possible further health-related issues in this population. Furthermore, the literature does not discuss timelines for pressure ulcer treatments and interventions related to casualties.

In addition to the absence of literature to guide pressure ulcer prevention and treatment, some practical considerations were related to the military. The accepted practice among health care facilities in the Department of Defense is to use the Braden Scale to assess which patients are at risk of developing pressure ulcers. The authors wondered if this is the gold standard in other health care systems. They identified two problems specific to the military that complicate decision making related to assessing pressure ulcers, determining risk factors, preventing pressure ulcers, and initiating nursing interventions in patients who are casualties from OIF and OEF. First, no established standards exist for determining which intervention should be used in the field setting or hospital. Second, the number of injuries that occur during armed conflicts makes it challenging to set realistic benchmarks (incidences per 1000 discharges) related to pressure ulcers.

DEVELOPMENT OF AN EVIDENCE-BASED PRESSURE ULCER PREVENTION AND INITIAL RISK ASSESSMENT TOOL FOR RETURNING MILITARY CASUALTIES

After review of the NNMC process for pressure ulcer prevention and management, it was noted that the current practice manual, which was initiated in 2004, was based on current best-practice evidence. An in-depth review indicated that NNMC was, in fact, in compliance with the IHI's "Getting Started Kit: Prevent Pressure Ulcers How-to Guide."[9] NNMC procedures included all "Six Essential Elements of Pressure Ulcer Prevention" identified in the IHI guideline:

1. Conduct a pressure ulcer admission assessment for all patients
2. Reassess risk for all patients daily
3. Inspect skin daily
4. Manage moisture: keep the patient dry and moisturize skin
5. Optimize nutrition and hydration
6. Minimize pressure.

At that point, further evaluation was justified because the implementation of a new guideline would not generate positive results if it were no different from the current process already in place. With the assistance of the hospital patient safety department, NNMC conducted a Failure Mode and Effect Analysis (FMEA) of the current process. An FMEA is an examination of an entire process to identify and rank the modes of failure within that process. Even though the pressure ulcer prevention process was in accordance with the current best practice, NNMC was experiencing an increased pressure ulcer rate, and the authors hypothesized that failure was occurring at some unidentified point or points within the process.

Identifying the source of the problem was the task of the FMEA group, which comprised members from throughout the facility who were familiar with the current pressure ulcer prevention and management process, and who were directly involved in patient care. Approximately 10 members began to look at this increase in pressure ulcer development. Group representation included nurses and health care technicians from all inpatient care units, a certified wound care nurse, the hospital Senior Nurse Executive, and a physician champion from the trauma service and surgical directorate. A patient safety representative skilled in using the FMEA process facilitated the group. The group reviewed the entire pressure ulcer prevention and management process, identifying and ranking critical elements within the process that, if not performed, would cause the entire process to fail. The outcome of the FMEA indicated that a mix of communication, documentation, and education issues was the root cause of the problem.

For pressure ulcer prevention among young military casualties, one of the most crucial elements is the accurate and timely completion of a pressure ulcer risk assessment tool to identify patients at high risk. The clinically validated Braden Scale for Predicting Pressure Sore Risk is the most commonly used standard tool for identifying and quantifying the severity of risk for pressure ulcer development. The Braden Scale has been, and remains, the tool used at many military facilities to quantify risk for pressure ulcer development in patients. The FMEA group noted that the Braden Scale was initiated on admission and performed at each shift, thus satisfying the first two essential elements of assessing pressure ulcer risk on admission, and reassessing daily.

However, despite an assessment being performed, nursing interventions were not always implemented, nor were they always based on the risk level identified. As a result of this finding, a comprehensive Nursing Practice Manual was developed to assist unit nurses.

EVIDENCE-BASED NURSING INTERVENTIONS

Managing moisture, keeping patients dry, and moisturizing their skin effectively were found to be common practice among nurses, and therefore no failure mode was identified. Patient nutrition and hydration were also being appropriately addressed in most instances by nurses, physicians, and nutrition care staff and did not pose a concern. Therefore, the source of the problem lay elsewhere in the nursing practices for pressure ulcer prevention and management.

Accepted nursing solutions to effectively minimize pressure are: (1) repositioning/turning the patient every 2 hours, (2) using heel protectors and heel elevation, (3) keeping the head of the bed at less than 30° if not contraindicated, (4) using cushions to relieve pressure to bony prominences, and, in extreme cases (5) relying on specialty mattresses that use air, foam, fluid, or gel to redistribute pressure over larger areas.[1] A review of nursing practices at NNMC indicated that not all of these solutions were being used. The most apparent problem was the nurses' overuse and dependence on specialty beds and mattresses. From October 2006 to September 2007, the cost for using specialty mattresses increased by approximately $80,000 from the previous 12 months. During the same timeframe, however, pressure ulcer incidence increased.

A more in-depth review identified a common misconception among nursing staff. Nurses believed that patients on a specialty bed or mattress did not need to be routinely turned or repositioned. The problem was compounded by the increased use of specialty beds for pulmonary management. Although these devices rotate the patient to assist in the prevention of pulmonary complications, the rotation is not designed to replace repositioning of the patient for pressure ulcer prevention. Another misconception was the use of the "turn assist" mode on a specialty mattress that allowed nurses to maintain patients in a side-lying position. The "turn assist" mode hyperinflates one side of the mattress to assist the caregiver in turning the patient to the opposite side. Once the patient has been turned and repositioned, the turn assist mode should be discontinued. Nurses erroneously believed they could leave the bed in the turn assist mode.

Another, and probably the most significant, finding is the conflicting information between pressure ulcer prevention and management recommendations and the IHI's "Getting Started Kit: Prevent Ventilator-Associated Pneumonia (VAP) How-to Guide" or VAP bundle. The VAP bundle is a series of interventions grouped together and designed to reduce the incidence of ventilator-associated pneumonia. The VAP guideline recommends that the head of the bed be placed at 30° to 45°.[9] However, the Wound Ostomy and Continence Nurses Society's "Guideline for Prevention and

Management of Pressure Ulcers"[10] recommends the head of the bed be placed at less than 30°. However, some service members require both ventilation and pressure ulcer prevention, depending on the severity of their injuries sustained in armed conflict. Either guideline alone can help health care providers provide evidence-based care, but the real issue is deciding when patients require both interventions. Currently, no connection between an increase in pressure ulcer incidence and the implementation of the VAP bundle is confirmed. However, the period during which the VAP bundle was successfully implemented coincided with the period during which the increase in pressure ulcer incidence was identified.

To identify additional problem areas, a thorough review of records from October 2007 to September 2008 was initiated for all patients who developed a pressure ulcer. The findings indicated the type of patient at the NNMC most at risk for developing a pressure ulcer. The review indicated that, regardless of age, most patients who developed a pressure ulcer had impaired neurologic status, impaired sensation, or impaired mobility from their related injury. These injuries include polytrauma injuries and traumatic brain injury. The neurologic, sensory, or mobility impairment was associated with either a brain or spinal cord injury, loss of sensation related to peripheral neuropathy, or impaired sensation from sedation, such as with ventilated patients.

IMPLEMENTING AN ELECTRONIC DOCUMENTATION/WOUND FLOW SHEET

The nursing admission and daily nursing assessment note located within the skin assessment section lacked detail and did not address pressure ulcer needs. Furthermore, because the skin assessment was located within the nursing notes, other health care providers (ie, physicians) had difficulty locating and reading the nurse's daily findings, leading to a breakdown in communication between nursing and physician providers when skin care issues arose. In addition, appropriate interventions were not always implemented or documented when a problem or risk was identified on the skin assessment.

The authors also noted a discrepancy in documentation among health care team members resulting from their varying practices and knowledge of pressure ulcer prevention. For example, the staging of a pressure ulcer was not always the same among nurses and providers, even on the same patient. This incongruity was identified in areas such as basic skin care, wound care, support surface selection, and patient need for repositioning. Pressure ulcer and wound care documentation occurred within daily nursing notes, making this information difficult to locate. Furthermore, with no standardized fields for documentation, charting and terminology was inconsistent among providers.

A Wound and Skin Care Flow Sheet was developed with the assistance of the information technology department (**Fig. 3**). This flow sheet was designed to facilitate communication among nurses and providers concerning pressure ulcer/skin and wound care interventions and treatments, wound healing, and characteristics of the wound. Drop down boxes and suggested responses helped standardize and educate personnel on the most pertinent information.

ESTABLISHMENT OF A WOUND CARE NURSE SPECIALIST

The authors' evaluation led them to realize the significance of NNMC's lack of a wound care specialty trained nurse. A dedicated nurse wound care specialist with a critical care background became a necessity at NNMC for returning OIF/OEF service members for several reasons. The nature of the injuries was severe

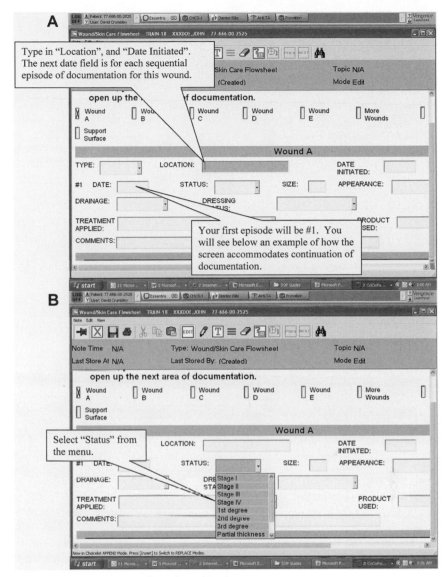

Fig. 3. Wound and skin care flow sheet (*A, B*).

and very complex, with many cases of polytrauma. These patients required ventilator support, needed head-of-bed elevation, had various orthopedic hardware and tubes, and had positioning requirements to reduce intracranial pressure. Thus, pressure ulcer prevention became paramount, but complicated. NNMC had a dedicated position for a wound care nurse, but unfortunately the position was vacant from April 2006 until early 2007.

New responsibilities of the wound care nurse were developed, such as providing consultation for advanced wound care patients, orienting new personnel, and

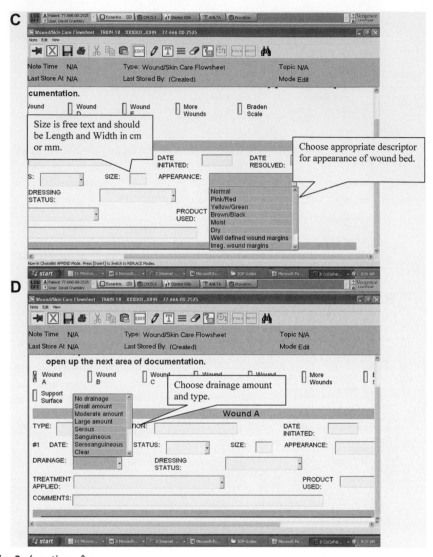

Fig. 3. (*continued*)

periodically training existing staff about pressure ulcer prevention and management, including specialty bed selection. Because the position was vacant for such a long time, employees and military nurses who arrived during 2006 did not benefit from the new orientation by the wound care nurse. This issue is particularly significant for a military facility because military staff move to new locations every 2 to 3 years. In addition, because of the conflicts in Iraq and Afghanistan, military staff members are also deployed to those areas for 6 months to 1 year and consequently miss the latest information on pressure ulcer prevention and management. The lack of timely training by the wound care nurse was therefore noticeable at first as the military staff (not trained in 2006) rotated to their locations

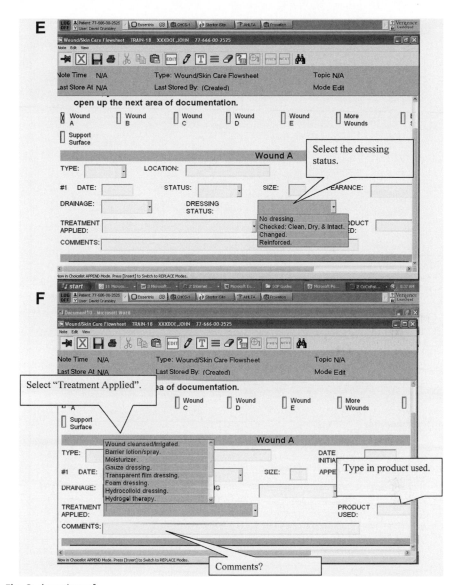

Fig. 3. (continued)

or were deployed. Training became paramount to the success of the pressure ulcer prevention program at NNMC.

NEED FOR COLLABORATION WITH OTHER SERVICES

Collaboration among all services—Army, Air Force, Navy, and Nurse Corps—was identified as a necessity for successfully preventing pressure ulcers in wounded service members. Members at NNMC worked closely with members of the Air Force and Army to successfully choose the right surface for the litters being used in patient air evacuations. Pressure ulcer prevention begins when the patients are being moved

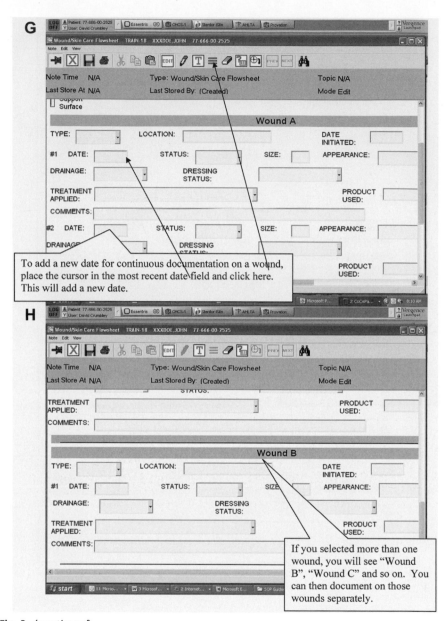

Fig. 3. (*continued*)

during their air transport from the battlefield to Germany and from Germany to the United States, and surface selection of the litters during air evacuation is the first critical step.

Members at NNMC also interfaced with members of the Air Force MedEvac process involved with surface selection during evacuation. One subject matter expert consulted was COL Elizabeth Bridges, USAF NC, who completed extensive research and evaluation of various support surfaces used during MedEvac and has extensive knowledge in this area.[5] Collaboration among these experts identified additional concerns needing further development to achieve a successful pressure ulcer program:

- Education concerning pressure ulcer assessment
- Improved pressure ulcer documentation
- Education concerning appropriate pressure ulcer prevention interventions
  - Techniques for positioning and repositioning
  - Education on preventing pressure ulcers in critically ill patients (ventilated or spinal cord injury)
  - Skin care education
  - Support surface selection and use of specialty beds
- Education on which patients are at highest risk
- Development of an approach to care that involves the patient's family members.

Pressure Ulcer Education as the Cornerstone to Pressure Ulcer Prevention

Practices were not standardized among nurses and providers regarding pressure ulcer assessment, treatment, and documentation. The solution was to add a section in the organization's pressure ulcer prevention procedure manual that visually identified the six pressure ulcer stages. The authors created concise Pressure Ulcer "Cliff's Notes" (**Fig. 4**), concentrating on three key interventions: (1) risk assessment with daily skin inspection and identification of high-risk patients, (2) moisture management, and (3) minimization of pressure through positioning and selection of pressure redistribution surfaces. These "Cliff's Notes" were transferred onto handouts and posters and placed in all patient care areas (see **Fig. 4**).

In addition, the group began educating incoming personnel, both nurses and physicians, assigned to NNMC. Didactic education of pressure ulcer prevalence

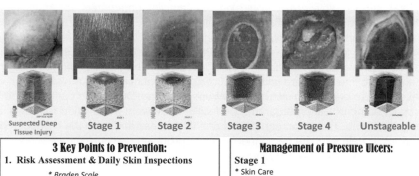

| Suspected Deep Tissue Injury | Stage 1 | Stage 2 | Stage 3 | Stage 4 | Unstageable |

3 Key Points to Prevention:	**Management of Pressure Ulcers:**
1. **Risk Assessment & Daily Skin Inspections**	**Stage 1**
* *Braden Scale*	* Skin Care
* *Inspect "from head to toe"*	* Off-Loading
2. **Moisture Management**	**Stage 2**
* *Keep skin DRY from bodily fluids*	* Off-Loading/Consider Specialty Bed
* *Moisturize and Protect skin*	* Use hydrocolloid or barrier cream for protection
3. **Minimization of Pressure**	**Stage 3**
* *Turn/reposition Q 2 hours*	* Consult Wound Care Nurse
* *Use pressure relieving surfaces*	* Order Specialty Bed
	* Appropriate Dressing
	Stage 4
High Risk Patients: Braden Scale <12, Elderly & Frail, Immobile, Spinal Cord Injury, TBI, Ventilator Dependent, Sensory Deficit(Epidural/Nerve Block), Sensory Neuropathy (Diabetic)	* Consult Wound Care Nurse
	* Maintain Specialty Bed
	* Consider Surgical vs. Non Surgical treatments

Fig. 4. Pressure ulcer prevention and management notes.

was integrated into the nursing orientation and preceptor courses. This educational program taught providers how to accurately identify and stage pressure ulcers. The directors of the various service areas were supportive and invited the pressure ulcer prevention team to speak to the Board of Directors (administrative and clinical) to discuss problems and potential solutions to this medical issue. Furthermore, the team discussed with physicians the need to identify and document pressure ulcers that are present on admission. This point became an issue during the chart review because the reviewers often were unable to distinguish between pressure ulcers present on admission and those that were hospital-acquired.

As a result of the chart reviews, the wound care nurse for NNMC presented on the topic of staging and documentation of pressure ulcers as part of the physician intern orientation program to enable these graduate medical officers to develop clinically sound skin assessment skills early in their educational training at NNMC.

The pressure ulcer prevention education component of the EBP project focused on the findings from the FMEA to eliminate the points of failure where education was crucial. Pressure ulcer prevention education led by the wound care team and the clinical nurse specialist group occurred throughout the facility. Education occurred in all inpatient areas, including the surgical procedure sections of the facility. Many of the wounded were undergoing repeated surgical procedures, placing them at risk for iatrogenic pressure ulcers. Nursing interns attended pressure ulcer prevention and skin care workshops as part of their training program.

In the intensive care area, education targeted preventing pressure ulcers in a high-risk population. Much discussion focused on repositioning critically ill patients (eg, those on a ventilator or brain injured) who could decompensate if repositioned, and identifying when a patient was decompensating. This solution required collaboration with the physician staff and resulted in improved physician–nurse communication. Previously, nurses in the intensive care unit were hesitant to reposition a critically ill patient because they were unsure whether this process would cause harm. The solution was simple: physicians would provide activity parameters for repositioning patients on a ventilator or who had a brain or spinal cord injury, thereby reducing the nurse's apprehension about positioning.

Another topic for the intensive care unit area, and other areas throughout the facility, was how to prevent incontinence-induced dermatitis in this population. Because most patients in the intensive care unit are critically ill, incontinence and moisture management are key to preventing skin damage from occurring. During this period, as part of a product standardization program, the facility underwent a transition to a new skin care product line. The group capitalized on this process and used the product representatives to help educate personnel on the appropriate use of skin care products to minimize skin damage from moisture and incontinence.

SUMMARY

The outcomes of the EBP project have been favorable. Since 2008, the educational efforts and presentations to physician and nursing groups have increased health care provider awareness of the pressure ulcer prevention process, improved pressure ulcer documentation and communication among nursing staff, and facilitated a team approach to pressure ulcer prevention and management. These accomplishments have contributed to a decrease in the incidence of pressure ulcers among wounded service members, particularly those in the 18- to 35-year-old age group. Facility expenditures for support surfaces and specialty mattresses decreased by more than $100,000 during the authors' focused educational effort concerning the appropriate use of specialty mattresses (this effort began before the rollout of the pressure ulcer prevention EBP project). This pressure ulcer prevention EBP project officially began in November 2008. At the end of the first quarter of 2009 (October through December, 2008), the pressure ulcer rate had decreased 20%. By March of 2009, the pressure ulcer rate at NNMC was at 27 incidences per 1000 discharges and almost at the AHRQ benchmark goal of 25 incidences per 1000 discharges. Further review found that the incidence rate would have been more favorable had "present on admission" pressure ulcers been better documented. However, the most significant finding concerned occurrences of stage III or IV pressure ulcers in the wounded population: none were documented after the implementation of this EBP project. All members of the health care team attribute this improvement in patient management to early assessment, recognition, and intervention to prevent worsening of pressure ulcers.

The increasing propensity for pressure ulcer development in the young military population, as a result of new weapon systems and use of IEDs, creates the possibility of wounds and pressure ulcer development, the health effects and toxicity characteristics of which have not been fully investigated, if at all. Standard pressure ulcer assessment tools alone do not meet the needs of these young casualties, nor are they enough to decrease the incidence and prevalence of pressure ulcers in combat casualties. A comprehensive assessment, risk factor identification, nursing intervention, and education program is warranted to balance the risk for more damage to surrounding tissue that could adversely affect the normal functioning of muscle and tissues.

This article highlights the importance of an evidence-based pressure ulcer program that uses nursing interventions, a documentation tool, a specialized wound care nurse, and a new wound care assessment system to rapidly assess and treat potential pressure ulcers. The implication to nursing science is twofold: (1) the systematic pressure ulcer prevention program developed at NNMC could be generalized and adapted by any MTF that receives OIF/OEF patients, and (2) the methodology of EBP, nursing assessment, interventions, and documentation has provided fundamental insights and useful baseline data that are being used to improve treatment and care of young veterans. The development of a comprehensive pressure ulcer program tailored to a specific population with polytrauma injuries is an important advance in military nursing.

REFERENCES

1. European Pressure Ulcer Advisory Panel and National Pressure Ulcer Advisory Panel. Prevention and treatment of pressure ulcers: quick reference guide. Washington, DC: National Pressure Ulcer Advisory Panel; 2009. Available at: http://www.npuap.org/Final_Quick_Prevention_for_web.pdf. Retrieved on December 14, 2009. Accessed September 12, 2009.
2. Levine J. Historical notes on pressure ulcers: the cure of Ambrose Pare. Decubitus 1992;5:23–4.
3. Munro D. Rehabilitation of veterans paralyzed as the result of injury to the spinal cord and cauda equina. Am J Surg 1948;75:3–18.
4. Thomas DR. Issues and dilemmas in the prevention and treatment of pressure ulcers: a review. J Gerontol A Biol Sci Med Sci 2001;56(6):M328–40.
5. Bridges EJ, Schmelz JO, Mazer S. Skin interface pressure on the NATO litter. Mil Med 2003;168(4):280–6.

6. AHRQ. Patient safety quality indicators. Available at: http://qualityindicators.ahrq.gov/downloads/psi/psi_provider_comparative_v31.pdf. Accessed September 12, 2009.
7. Institute for Healthcare Improvement. Getting started kit: prevent pressure ulcers how-to guide. 5 Million Lives Campaign. Cambridge (MA): Institute for Healthcare Improvement; 2008.
8. Harrow JJ, Rashka SL, Fitzgerald SG, et al. Pressure ulcers and occipital alopecia in Operation Iraqi Freedom polytrauma casualties. Mil Med 2008; 173(11):1068–72.
9. Campaign ML. Getting started kit: prevent ventilator-associated pneumonia how-to guide. Cambridge (MA): Institute for Healthcare Improvement; 2008.
10. Wound, Ostomy and Continence Nurses Society. Guideline for prevention and management of pressure ulcers. WOCN clinical practice guideline series. Glenview (IL): WOCN; 2003.

Military Nursing Competencies

Mary Candice Ross, PhD, RN

KEYWORDS

• Military • Nursing • Competency • Skills • War

Providing nursing care to a Marine in a blinding dust storm was a test of my endurance as well as my clinical skills. We were inside a tent, but the tent sides were flapping so loudly that the sounds in my stethoscope were meaningless. My assessment of his tissue perfusion relied on my astute observation of his skin color, capillary refill, and level of consciousness. It could only have been worse if this day in the desert had included chemical warfare gear!
    Air Force Nurse, Iraq, 2006

Thousands of military nurses have moved into the civilian nursing workforce over the past decade. All bring unique military skills with them. The array of abilities military nurses acquire during their careers can be organized by three sets of competencies: patient care, deployment, and leadership. After providing a general overview of military nurses, I offer a brief look at each of these competency sets.

GENERAL CHARACTERISTICS OF MILITARY NURSES

The military is a broad term that encompasses the Army, Navy, Air Force, and Marines. Military nurses provide care for all four branches, but because health care for the Navy and Marines is combined, nurses themselves serve in the Army, Navy, or Air Force. Nurses from each service have particular areas of responsibility when they are deployed to a war zone or a humanitarian mission. The Army Nurse Corps is the oldest of the three nurse corps and Army nurses are trained to work primarily near the battlefront in portable hospitals and clinics to care for casualties close to the conflict or disaster. Navy nurses are trained to work from ships and to support the transport of the injured from battle areas to ports or flight lines. Air Force nurses are primarily responsible for transporting patients to fixed hospitals for more definitive care. When they are not deployed, nurses from all three services practice in stateside and overseas hospitals and clinics, providing care to individuals injured on the battlefield or in a disaster as well as military beneficiaries (families and retired service members).

College of Nursing, Florida State University, PO Box 3064310, Tallahassee, FL 32306-4310, USA
E-mail address: cross3@fsu.edu

Nurs Clin N Am 45 (2010) 169–177
doi:10.1016/j.cnur.2010.02.006
0029-6465/10/$ – see front matter © 2010 Elsevier Inc. All rights reserved.

nursing.theclinics.com

All three branches of the military use a variety of nursing personnel ranging from registered nurses to medics and independent duty corpsmen. The medics and independent duty corpsmen are enlisted personnel who undergo rigorous training that provides them with sophisticated skill sets to deal with battlefield injuries. Although many of the nursing personnel who work in military hospitals are career civilian employees or contract workers, and not members of the military, this article focuses on RNs who are in the military's active and reserve forces and describes their unique nursing role.

The primary responsibilities of all military nurses are their military obligations.[1] All RNs become "officers" when they join the military, adding a dimension to their job duties that differentiates them from civilian RNs. At present, regardless of the branch of service, as a requirement for joining the military, nurses must have graduated from an accredited baccalaureate program and have successfully completed the same licensing examination as their civilian counterparts. As military officers, their pay is commensurate with rank and is the same across the branches of service. The rank designations of the Army and Air Force are the same, starting with second lieutenant (O-1) and going through colonel (O-6). The Navy ranks are different in that the entry rank (O-1) is ensign and the typical senior level rank (O-6) is captain. Nurse Corps officers are promoted according to their years of experience, education, and performance reviews. Each of the Army, Navy, and Air Force Corps are directed by a general officer such as a Corps Chief. Ancillary nursing personnel such as nursing assistants or licensed practical nurses are "enlisted" and commonly referred to as corpsmen. They have ranks such as sergeant or petty officer and are trained to varying levels of skill—from providing first aid to becoming licensed practical nurses.

Many nurses are commissioned into the military directly from their schooling, but some entering nurses have years of work experience and bring an array of valued experiences with them when they are sworn in as military officers. Unlike most civilian nurses, military nurses of all three services have a career development plan that is used to guide their assignments. Beginning as staff nurses to acquire clinical expertise, military nurses move into positions with increased responsibilities as they advance in rank. Because military nurses relocate to new geographic areas every 2 to 3 years, they must be flexible and adaptable, learning to quickly assess new situations and accommodate to new ways of doing things. A pervasive principle is that the military nurse is expected to continue developing new knowledge and skills with advancing rank and responsibilities. Consequently, the military affords nurses an assortment of experiences and career opportunities not typically found among their civilian counterparts, ranging from hospital direct care, trauma nurse coordinators,[2] leadership positions, case managers,[3] nurse practitioners, nurse educators, nurse anesthetists, to first responders. Each specialty has a set of competencies that may be prescribed by regulations, operating instructions (procedural requirements), or service guidelines. These competencies are acquired in a variety of ways—from on-the-job training, to graduate education at a civilian university, to training at military specialty schools.

Beyond the basic skills and hospital orientation common to the training of all nurses, military nurses participate in operational readiness training and exercises to test their ability to respond to a disaster or wartime patient surge, joint readiness exercises to practice the interface with other military services, and mass casualty drills with civilian facilities. Operational readiness pertains to preparing the hospital or medical treatment facility to receive combat or disaster casualties or respond to terrorist threats. Joint readiness refers to the military interface between the Army, Navy, and Air Force and even allied foreign military forces to respond to a regional or national threat.

Nurses are expected to be familiar with an immense number of military terms and processes, and to be proficient in processing patients among the services without care delays or losing equipment along the way. For example, just ensuring that you can replace the respirator that goes out with a trauma patient can be critical when you are expecting further casualties on the same day.

The interface between military and civilian agencies requires knowledge about protecting military confidential, classified, or secret information. Beginning with officer's training, nurses are thoroughly informed about the risks of disclosing sensitive information. They must avoid revealing information that, if it made its way into enemy hands, could be used against the United States. For instance, to maintain national security, military nurses learn to guard the numbers, job responsibilities, and locations of personnel. Even casual conversations during a social interaction with nonmilitary individuals must be conducted with considerations of how seemingly insignificant information could result in a breech of confidentiality.

For practicing military nurses, critical thinking, clinical competence, and knowledge of military triage are fundamental demands.[4] Critical thinking is most essential for military nurses because they are expected to make decisions in environments where time, resources, and consultation are scarce. Military triage differs from civilian triage in that the objective is to determine which service members can return to duty immediately and which need treatment. A policy is established for each conflict or battlefield situation that dictates how quickly injured military personnel will be moved for more definitive care. In practice, this means that the nurse knows how the patient is to be triaged and treated. If the evacuation policy is "immediate," the patient may be stabilized for urgent transport to definitive hospital care. Some service members may be stabilized and then wait several days for evacuation if the conflict is more remote. In these cases, only the most life-threatening cases will be transported immediately.

NURSING COMPETENCIES

Along with expected competencies in basic nursing skills and professional practice, the competencies that distinguish military nurses are those related to the unique care requirements of the military patient populations, deployment of nursing personnel and equipment, and leadership. Each of these areas of competency is developed within service-specific knowledge and skills (**Table 1**). The Army, Navy, and Air Force each use their own prescribed process and format for annotating military competencies, called a training record. Through a system of mentoring and evaluating proficiency in important skills and knowledge, the competencies of each nurse are periodically reviewed and the nurse's training record is updated.

PATIENT CARE COMPETENCIES

The patient population for military nurses is incredibly broad and subject to change on a moment's notice, making it necessary for these caregivers to have an exceptionally wide range of abilities. In contrast to most civilian nurses, the military nurse must develop skills in caring for severely injured, multitrauma, combat victims. For instance, a military nurse who works in labor and delivery must also be ready to deploy to a combat zone, live in austere conditions, and provide care in extraordinary circumstances, such as to starving families who are victims of a famine or to burned soldiers on a ship in the Persian Gulf.

In addition to the military nurse's general preparedness for patient care, each branch of the military service has its own unique nursing roles that demand high proficiency in a distinct set of competencies. Air Force flight nurses, for example, set up

Table 1	
Examples of unique military nurse corps competencies	
Competency Category	**Knowledge or Skill**
Nursing practice	Ability to provide care for seriously injured combat or trauma patients Knowledge of battlefield, multitrauma injuries Ability to treat victims of chemical, biological, or radiological terrorism
Military service	Knowledge of military mission Ability to interact according to military protocols Knowledge of military regulations Skills for patient movement from battlefield to stateside definitive care Knowledge of survival skills
Leadership	Supervision of a variety of enlisted personnel Ability to motivate personnel in high-stress environments Personal skill in stress management

facilities and provide care in fixed-wing cargo aircraft. Military aircraft have multipurpose designs so that an airplane that drops paratroopers or hauls cargo can be converted by nurses and medical technicians to carry patients. There is no equivalent civilian nursing role. The Air Force provides formal education programs for flight nurses and requires further qualification practice training on the ground and on flights. Competency "check-rides" are also required periodically for flight nurses to maintain their qualification.

Army nurses also transport patients in a variety of aircraft and vehicles, including helicopters and ground personnel carriers. These nurses have skills in setting up and providing care for patients in tents or other improvised hospitals where there may not be much protection from the outside environment and where asepsis can be a challenge to achieve. Murdock[5] described the deployed environments for Army nurses as being characterized by "austere and dangerous conditions, high patient variability, and limited technology."

Navy nurses must develop skills specific to providing care on cramped ships and moving casualties between helicopters and aircraft. Navy nurses are often the first to receive patients with battle injuries who come by helicopter to the ship. Aboard ship, it is routine for just one nurse to provide preventative and routine health care and first aid to thousands of seamen.

DEPLOYMENT COMPETENCIES

Military nursing practice is based on the premise that the nurse will be ready to mobilize to a stateside location or deploy overseas on short notice. This competency is called deployment readiness. Military nurses train to be ready for deployments associated with low- or high-intensity conflicts, peacekeeping missions, or disaster relief. Low-intensity conflicts are faced every day by nurses assigned overseas where sniper or terrorist attacks are likely. High-intensity conflicts include war zones where numerous casualties need care. Deployment competencies include the ability to provide complex patient care in a hostile environment, sometimes with very limited resources and often with makeshift equipment. Skills in the use of chemical/biological protection and the use of special deployment equipment, such as mobile hospitals, tents, and patient transport devices, are also a part of deployment readiness training.

Providing nursing care while wearing protective gear means trying to "see" the pulse in an unprotected patient when you cannot feel it through the heavy rubber gloves that are a part of the protective garb. It is also a challenge to work for an extended period of time perspiring heavily under a chemical suit with that "Darth Vader" breathing sound in your ears—a sound created by the full-hooded head gear that has goggles to look through and a respirator to breathe through.

Deployment competencies encompass a wide array of performance skills depending on the nurse's branch of military service and nursing role or job category. The deployment briefing that precedes departure usually includes information about cultural precautions as well as the environmental hazards to be expected. Deployment readiness includes a special process to check everything from essential uniforms, to wills, dog tags, immunizations, chemical protective gear, and survival equipment. Specialty nurses, such as flight nurses and nurse anesthetists, also have lists of items that cannot be left behind such as personal oxygen masks, flight checklists, and special medical equipment.

Although most military nurses are serving in hospitals and clinics in the United States, deployments of 3 to 12 months send nurses to foreign locations such as Japan, Korea, Germany, Iraq, and Afghanistan. The military nursing in the hospitals and clinics of Japan or Germany could be similar to military stateside duties; however, these locations may also be the first definitive hospital care for multitrauma patients flown from Afghanistan or Iraq. Deployments often put military nurses in a practice environment that presents cultural challenges. Military nursing practice includes interacting with civilians, foreign military, and medical personnel from outside the United States. In-depth understanding of local cultures is essential for effective communication when interacting with individuals in other countries. Differences in personal freedoms, legal authorities, health beliefs, and human rights can have a significant impact on patient care and nursing practice.[6] For example, if a female military nurse needs to talk to Iraqi military personnel about preparing for transferring patients from a helicopter to a plane, she may need to take a male military person with her to do the direct communication because the foreign national may not be willing to interact with a woman. It may also be critical to avoid direct eye contact and even to wear an abaya over her uniform to avoid a cultural insult or unwanted advances. Different regions of countries have their own unique customs that need to be reviewed so a military nurse can be prepared to work effectively.

Cultural competency for military nursing goes beyond the usual interface with patients of different ethnicities. It includes skills related to the differences among the three military services that can facilitate or obstruct interservice systems for patient movement. For example, the Army may use one type of patient ventilator while the Air Force uses another, requiring a change-out of equipment as a patient transfers from an Army hospital in the war zone to an Air Force aircraft for evacuation. Other features of military cultural competency include personal safety, protection from extreme environmental hazards, chemical- and biological-threat protection, and troop movement logistics. Each service may have differing but equally safe protective gear or different methods for employing protective postures. This becomes important as Air Force or Navy nurses are deployed to Army facilities and visa versa.

LEADERSHIP COMPETENCIES

Military nurses have assumed an increasing number of health care manager and leadership positions that have not traditionally been assigned to nurses. Army nurses are increasingly being assigned to what are called branch immaterial positions such as company commander, policy development, career development, leadership of combat support hospitals, and hospital executive officers. Air Force Flight Nurses are becoming Aeromedical Evacuation Unit commanders responsible for radio communications personnel, medical administrators, and even large inventories of vehicles. Expanded leadership roles for nurses have increased the demand for greater competency in finance management, information technology, data analysis, personnel management, and organizational change. Leadership among military nurses is often considered a given because the nurse is an officer, and having that status implies being a leader. The military, however, sees leadership as something that should be taught to new Nurse Corps officers. It begins with Basic Training, an orientation to wearing the uniform properly, saluting, marching, and generally becoming familiar with military acronyms, policies, and way of life. A central feature of the officers' orientation course is an emphasis on the responsibilities of leadership. Leadership is integral to military nursing. Even as staff nurses, along with their patient care responsibilities, Nurse Corps officers supervise multiple enlisted personnel who are part of the care team in military hospitals. Throughout their careers, military nurses are expected to advance their leadership knowledge and skills through formal military schools, training, special exercises for emergencies, mentored experiences, and other development activities. Assignments are made to afford each Nurse Corps officer progressive leadership responsibilities. Graduate education is regarded as a part of leadership development. Consequently, the Army, Navy, and Air Force Nurse Corps each sponsor programs that allow individuals to apply for competitive selection master's or doctoral degree programs. The nurses selected for this opportunity are given paid leave to attend school.

Because leadership is central to a military career, there is an ongoing interest in identifying leadership competencies to ensure that military officers, including nurses, develop these competencies. For example, to fulfill the requirements for a master's degree in an Army-sponsored Health Care Administration program, a Delphi study was done involving 200 senior Navy nurses to identify leadership competencies in Navy nurse executives (**Table 2**).[7] The top ranked leadership knowledge, skills, and abilities pertained to integrity, communication skills, mentoring, active listening, holding people accountable, interpersonal skills, team-building, and the ability to lead and manage change. An interesting contrast between leadership for military and civilian positions can be found in these data. The competencies that were ranked the lowest by the Navy nurses related to business management, a mainstay in civilian leadership and management positions. Conversely, global awareness, or an understanding of the interrelatedness of multiple cultural perspectives, was a requisite skill for Navy nurse executives.[7] This domain is not listed among competencies for civilian nurse leaders.

Leadership is expected from all military nurses, not just those at the executive level. For example, leadership is an essential feature of nurses' readiness to deploy.[8] All military nurses need leadership competencies to effectively lead hundreds of personnel who may be functioning in austere and possibly life-threatening situations. This level of leadership is unlike the demands of civilian nursing leadership positions in that it requires a high degree of personal resilience in an environment of potential "moral distress." Fry and colleagues[9] describe the phenomena of "moral distress" in military nursing as performing expert care in high-stress environments for extended time periods while at great risk of personal harm. The broad scope of practice and deployment arenas with the potential for mass casualties demands advanced skills in leadership among all military nurses.

Rank of Importance	Domain	Skills, Knowledge, or Abilities
Table 2 **Skills, knowledge, and abilities for Navy nurse executives**		
1	Executive leadership	Maintains the utmost integrity; has the trust of all members inside and outside of the organization
2	Professional development	Communication skills: ability to communicate in all forms
3	Professional development	Ability to lead and mentor junior personnel
4	Communications	Ability to actively listen
5	Professional development	Ability to hold all accountable for personal and professional actions
6	Communications	Ability to communicate across all levels of the health care continuum—from the perspective of the patient, nurse, health care organization, and business organization
7	Executive leadership	Communication skills
8	Communications	Interpersonal skills: connect with your people, know your people and your colleagues, and be forthright, which is different than being brutally honest
9	Executive leadership	Team building: collaborate with all disciplines as part of the health care team
10	Global awareness and interoperability	Ability to lead and manage change

From Palarca C, Johnson S, Mangelsdorff AD, et al. Building from within: identifying leadership competencies for future Navy nurse executives. Nurs Admin Q 2008;32:216–25; with permission.

COMPETENCY MEASUREMENT

Readiness is the term generally used to describe the level of preparation nurses have that enables them to fulfill their wartime and disaster-relief missions of patient care. Evaluation of readiness competency, along with ongoing training, is a basic paradigm of military nursing. Validation of military nursing readiness competencies has been conducted in several studies using the Readiness Estimate and Deployability Index (READI) instrument,[8] the Operational nursing competencies checklist,[10] and the Emergency Preparedness Information Questionnaire (EPIQ).[11] These instruments measure the competencies of military nurses to assess training needs as well as skill profiles. The dynamic nature of the military mission as well as the need to fight unpredictable tactics of terrorists makes consistent evaluation of knowledge and trauma skills a critical part of any military career development.

Franklin and colleagues[12] reported a study of trauma competencies among Army nurse practitioners. The self-assessment was based on 29 competencies taken from courses such as Advanced Trauma Life Support, Advanced Trauma Care for Nursing, and the Tactical Nursing Combat Casualty Course. Although the nurse practitioners who had prior intensive care or emergency department experience self-reported higher trauma competencies, in the aggregate, the nurse practitioners in the study perceived themselves as competent in trauma management,[12] though there was wide variance. This indicates the need for consistent training in trauma management before nurses are deployed.

Another area of competency for military nurses that requires routine reassessment is use of current military, medical, and information technology. Advancements in technology are not only brought to deployments, but they are also developed as a consequence of needs recognized during deployments. For example, the use of vacuum-assisted wound-closure devices, continuous peripheral nerve catheters, and synthetic blood are developments that many civilian nurses do not see on a regular basis but have become second nature to military nurses. In addition, military equipment and supplies must be evaluated for safety, effectiveness at high altitudes, use in extreme temperatures, long shelf life, disinfection or sterilization in austere environments, and portability for military use. Information technology is integral to care in deployed situations and therefore a requisite competency. Military patients are cared for and transported around the world on a daily basis. This necessitates a sophisticated system for patient tracking, electronic health records, and comprehensive personnel databases. For example, a Marine with polytrauma, including spinal cord injuries, may leave his unit in Iraq, receive initial care in Iraq at an Army field hospital, move by helicopter to a ship, and then be transported in a military aircraft to Germany. This same Marine may ultimately need all of his medical records with him at the Veteran's Administration hospital in Tampa, Florida, where service members with spinal cord injuries are undergoing rehabilitation. This interface between military and Veteran's Administration health care is essential to the seamless movement of trauma patients from the battlefield to their hometown; it also requires nurses to be competent in its use.

Nurses have assumed an increasing number of health care manager and leadership positions that have not traditionally been assigned to nurses. Army nurses are increasingly being assigned to what is called branch immaterial positions such as company commander, policy development, career development, leadership of combat support hospitals, and hospital executive officers. Air Force Flight Nurses are becoming Aeromedical Evacuation Unit commanders responsible for radio communications personnel, medical administrators, and even large inventories of vehicles. Expanded leadership roles for nurses have increased the demand for greater competency in finance management, information technology, data analysis, personnel management, and organizational change. Military nurses of the future will have a wider range of skills with the critical responsibility of protecting the fit force, treating injured warriors and their families, and caring for our military retirees.

SUMMARY

Military nurses practice in dynamic and demanding environments that may include deployments to austere and dangerous locations. Competencies for military nursing practice include skills for battlefield care of multitrauma patients, care in military vehicles and aircraft, mass casualty care, and military-specific skills. Leadership competencies are integral to every practice and specialty role in the military. The future of military nursing relies heavily on increasing abilities in leadership. Evaluation and research in military nursing competencies will contribute to the formulation of the best training and officer development for the demands of practice that range from providing care in up-to-date modern facilities to the battlefield and disaster settings. Military nurses of the future will have a wider range of skills with the critical responsibility of protecting the fit force, treating injured warriors and their families, and caring for our military retirees.

REFERENCES

1. Kraemer LC. A military twist to the profession of nursing. Medsurg Nurs 2008;17: 275–7.

2. Fecura SE, Martin C, Martin KD, et al. Nurse' role in the joint theater trauma system. J Trauma Nurs 2008;15:170–3.
3. Stanton MP, Swanson C, Baker RD. Development of a military competency checklist for case management. Lippincotts Case Manag 2005;10:128–35.
4. Bridges E. Wartime competencies for the USAF nurse: training for sustainment. Commun Nurs Res; 2006 Springfielder;39:365.
5. Murdock P. U.S. Army nursing readiness: a field administration of the Readiness Estimate and Deployability Index (READI) in the North Atlantic Regional Medical Command (NARMC). Academy of Health Sciences (Army) Fort Sam Houston TX Health Care Administration; TriService Nursing Research Program Final Report, 2001.
6. Spector R. Cultural diversity in health and illness. 4th edition. Stamford (CT): Appleton & Lange; 1996.
7. Palarca C, Johnson S, Mangelsdorff AD, et al. Building from within: identifying leadership competencies for future Navy nurse executives. Nurs Adm Q 2008; 32:216–25.
8. Reineck C, Finstuen K, Connelly LM, et al. Army nurse readiness instrument: psychometric evaluation and field administration. Mil Med 2001;166:931–9.
9. Fry ST, Harvey RM, Hurley AC, et al. Development of a model of moral distress in military nursing. Nurs Ethics 2002;9:373–87.
10. Bridges E. Combat casualty care: integrative review and validation of nursing competencies. Available at: http://www.son.washington.edu/research/grants/ShowAbstract.asp?Project. Accessed May 1, 2009.
11. Garbutt SJ, Peltier JW, Fitzpatrick J. Evaluation of an instrument to measure nurses' familiarity with emergency preparedness. Mil Med 2008;173:1073–7.
12. Franklin BE, Carr KV, Padden DL. Self-assessment of trauma competencies among Army family nurse practitioners. Mil Med 2008;173:759–64.

Uniformed Service Nurses' Experiences with the Severe Acute Respiratory Syndrome Outbreak and Response in Taiwan

Tsui-Lan Chou, MSN, RN[a], Li-Yuan Ho, MSN, RN[a],
Kwua-Yun Wang, PhD, RN[b,c], Chi-Wen Kao, PhD, RN[c],
Meei-Horng Yang, MSN, RN[d], Pao-Luo Fan, MMM, MD[e],*

KEYWORDS

- Uniformed service nurses • Military nursing • SARS outbreak
- Response • Taiwan

Severe Acute Respiratory Syndrome (SARS) began with an outbreak in Guangdong Province of mainland China in mid-November 2002. The epidemic almost immediately became a global crisis as it spread with lightning speed to places, such as Hong Kong, Canada, Singapore, and Vietnam. The rapid spread was primarily caused by advances in worldwide travel where the virus was carried by people via airplane. Frequent travel

The opinions or assertions contained herein are solely the views of the authors and should not be construed as official or reflecting the views of the Department of Defense or Taiwan Government.
[a] Nursing Department, Songshan Armed Forces General Hospital, No. 131, Jiankang Road, Songshan District, Taipei City 10581, Taiwan, Republic of China
[b] Nursing Department, Taipei Veterans General Hospital, No. 201, Sec. 2, Shipai Road, Taipei 11217, Taiwan, Republic of China
[c] School of Nursing, National Defense Medical Center, No. 161, Sec. 6, Min-Chuan East Road, Taipei 114, Taiwan, Republic of China
[d] Nursing Department, Wei-Gong Memorial Hospital, No. 128, Xinyi Road, Toufen Township, Miaoli County 351, Taiwan, Republic of China
[e] Medical Affairs Bureau, Ministry of National Defense, 3F., No. 164, Bo-Al Road, Taipei 10048, Taiwan, Republic of China
* Corresponding author.
E-mail address: h815200@ms25.hinet.net

between Taiwan and mainland China caused Taiwan to also became involved in this crisis.[1,2]

The first SARS case in Taiwan was discovered on March 14, 2003 when six employees from CTCI Corporation were infected with SARS while on a business trip to mainland China. Only then did the Taiwanese government begin to institute international epidemic prevention measures and take steps to isolate and quarantine those who wereinfected. However, those steps were not taken in time to prevent further outbreaks of nosocomial SARS infection in several Taiwanese hospitals. In total, there were 3021 suspected cases of SARS; 346 were confirmed and there were 73 deaths. Many more people were placed in home quarantine. There were two classes of home quarantine. The 50,319 individuals placed in Level A home quarantine had been in close contact with a patient with SARS and were quarantined for 10 to 14 days. Another 80,813 individuals were placed in Level B quarantine. These individuals were travelers arriving on flights from World Health Organization (WHO)-designated SARS-affected areas; they were quarantined for 10 days either at home, airport hotels, or government quarantine centers.[1] The events related to the SARS outbreak had an enormous impact on the public health and economy of Taiwan.[1] In this article, the authors describe the Taiwanese efforts to stem the spread of the disease and the role of Taiwan's military nurses during the epidemic. The authors discuss the public and private impact on the Taiwanese people and those military nurses who cared for patients with SARS or suspected SARS.

IMPACT OF SEVERE ACUTE RESPIRATORY SYNDROME ON TAIWAN'S SOCIETY

Although the first cases of SARS in Taiwan occurred in March, the first nosocomial case of SARS occurred in a hospital in Taipei city on April 24, 2003.[1] Continuous mass media reporting of the spread of the SARS epidemic created much fear and widespread hysteria among the people of Taiwan. At the beginning of the outbreak, SARS was an unknown infectious disease and the modes of transmission and methods of treatment were unclear. In addition, the mortality rate was also unknown. This lack of information had a significant impact on many aspects of the Taiwanese society, including health care, lifestyle, interpersonal interactions, education, and the economy of the country.

Health Care

Because of the threat of SARS, many patients were afraid to go to the hospital, even for reasons other than SARS-like symptoms. This resulted in a 51.6% decrease in emergency room visits,[3] and a 19.9% to 52.5% decrease in the number of in-patients[4] in hospitals across the country. Community residents were opposed to establishing SARS-dedicated clinics and SARS-dedicated hospitals in their locales. This opposition manifested itself in actions and words with local people blocking their roads to prevent the entry of patients with SARS. Waste disposal services refused to remove SARS medical wastes, creating a pile up of infectious materials. In addition, mortuary owners were reluctant to undertake those who had died of SARS for fear of contracting the disease themselves.[5]

Lifestyle and Interpersonal Interactions

At the beginning of the epidemic, the mode of SARS transmission was not known. People began to change their normal behaviors to include avoiding close contact with others, staying at home to minimize their interactions with others, wearing face-masks in confined spaces, greatly increasing the use of household disinfectant, measuring their body temperature every day, and isolating themselves if they had a fever. These changes had a critical impact on people's lifestyle, leisure activities, personal behaviors, social life, and interpersonal relationships. Societal perceptions toward the status and role of health care workers also changed during that time. First-line SARS health care workers, such as medical and nursing staff, were shunned by the community.

Education

School systems were also heavily affected by the SARS epidemic. The children of first-line SARS health care workers were asked not to attend primary and secondary schools. In addition, some parents kept their children home from school to minimize their chance of getting infected with SARS. At the university level, student nurses did not attend clinical practice in the hospitals during the SARS epidemic period.[1]

The Economy

The SARS epidemic had a direct and negative influence on the nation's financial stability. People in Taiwan stayed as close to home as possible to avoid getting infected. This isolation resulted in a large decline in commercial trading activities, greatly effecting Taiwan's economy, including manufacturing, commerce, the service industry, finance, and foreign investment. In addition, the epidemic had an undesirable effect on Taiwan's travel-related industries, such as tourism, transportation, hotel, and catering. As a result of declining tourism, sales decreased from of 10% to 90%.[6–8]

GOVERNMENT'S CONTROL MEASURES

To prevent the spread of the SARS epidemic and minimize its impact on the Taiwanese society, the government implemented strategies and interventions in an attempt to control the epidemic. These strategies included establishing a SARS-epidemic operation center by the Center for Disease Control, Republic of China (CDC, ROC), Department of Health on March 17, 2003. The purpose of this SARS center was to propose infection preventive interventions and health education advocacy.

On March 28, 2003, 4 months after its first appearance on mainland China, the CDC announced SARS as a new and previously unknown communicable disease. This recognition of SARS as a new communicable disease bolstered support to apply different epidemic preventative measures. Because of the seriousness of the epidemic, the Committee of SARS prevention, treatment, and bailout was also established on March 28, 2003.

The premier of Taiwan led the establishment of the SARS prevention and treatment policy. The interim regulations of SARS prevention, treatment, and bailout were announced by the president of Taiwan on May 2, 2003; they remained in effect until December 31, 2003. A total of 50 billion Taiwanese dollars (Approximately $1.5 billion) were allocated to cover all the required expenses requested by local governments for the management of SARS prevention, treatment, and bailout.[9]

Several measures were put into place to manage personnel entering and leaving the country. Prompt updates on epidemic source information were needed to prevent community-acquired SARS. Strict quarantine measures and isolation facilities were established to decrease the impact of diseases brought into the country and to strengthen quarantine management for potential isolated carriers. As previously noted, domestic, at-home isolation measures were instituted to avoid a wider spread of the epidemic. Individuals entering Taiwan from other epidemic regions were also quarantined. Living arrangements were made for those who were responsible for implementing isolation procedures. There was coordination with vendors to ensure an adequate supply of medical goods to care for isolated patients. Medical supply manufacturers were given assistance so they could improve their capacity to provide the supplies needed for treatment and prevention measures associated with the epidemic.

To effectively prevent the spread of SARS, epidemic-prevention measures were strongly emphasized. Hospitals dedicated solely to SARS were established in certain geographic areas for intensive treatment and an epidemic prevention Web site network for the public was constructed. Interventions of market and finance stabilization were adapted to provide bailout assistance for the industries that were adversely affected by the epidemic, and a fund was established to provide financial support for persons in quarantine.[1,10,11]

In coordination with the government's epidemic prevention policy, The Ministry of National Defense Republic of China established a "National Defense Emergency Response Team for SARS Prevention and Treatment." It also fully supported the government's epidemic prevention by mobilizing human and material resources. This mobilization included activating military medical resources and medical care manpower from the Medical Affairs Bureau, Ministry of National Defense. In addition, special troops were designated to support environmental chemical disinfection. In all, a total of 32,809 military personnel provided support during the epidemic. They contributed greatly toward SARS prevention in Taiwan. Local military barracks were even used to house health care workers working with isolated patients and to store first-line SARS preventive and health care products. Military personnel also intensively monitored the epidemic situation and the military troops providing care.[5]

ROLES AND FUNCTIONS OF THE MILITARY DURING THE SEVERE ACUTE RESPIRATORY SYNDROME OUTBREAK

Under the plan executed by Department of Health, Executive Yuan and the Ministry of National Defense, the SongShan Armed Forces Hospital received an emergency order from the Ministry of National Defense on the night of April 25, 2003 to immediately activate their crisis management plan. SongShan Armed Forces Hospital was officially designated to create the first isolation wards for receiving suspected SARS carriers from Ho-Ping Hospital. The hospital initiated an emergency call to all the military and civilian medical staff. The nursing department was given responsibility for planning the implementation of designated SARS wards and the patients' care. The nursing department immediately began to scrutinize the current operations and assess existing patients in all hospital wards. They arranged for next day discharge for patients whose conditions permitted them to leave the hospital. Those patients requiring continued hospitalization were transferred to specified wards.

On April 26, the designated SARS wards were completely vacated; they were cleaned, disinfected, and setup to receive patients with SARS. That same afternoon, SongShan Armed Forces Hospital and medical staff from the six municipal Taipei Hospitals discussed their planned mode of operation for these wards. The discussion focused on an integrated approach of the isolation wards' facilities, ventilation, protective interventions, and the priority of patients requiring more intense care. A decision was made to use the hospital's nursing care operation form as the key point record of nursing care histories. Admission of patients with SARS began in the early morning the next day.

To alleviate the severe epidemic situation in the northern region of Taiwan, on May 2, 2003, SongShan Armed Forces Hospital expanded its mission to become Taiwan's first dedicated hospital for day-care treatment of patients with SARS. The hospital set up 102 negative-pressure isolation rooms in the medical building. These included examination rooms, the operating room, intensive care center, dialysis room, delivery room, and the nursery. This action was taken to provide comprehensive management to the problems patients with SARS had. While the negative pressure system was constructed, the nursing staff was given education in the areas of SARS and its treatments and the nursing care standards that had been developed. Psychological counseling was also available for the staff to ease their anxiety associated with caring for patients with SARS. Staff working hours were minimized to reduce the physical load and the demands of working on the negative pressure wards.

Once the wards were cleaned and prepared for operation, the nursing department received the order to begin transferring or discharging patients. This order was communicated to the patients and their families, and on May 5, those patients who could safely go home were discharged and others were transferred. On May 21, the inpatients with SARS were admitted to the negative-pressure wards at SongShan for treatment. The rest of the 17 military hospitals in Taiwan were placed on standby, ready for the transfer of patients with SARS if necessary. This isolation measure was the most critical medical service provided for patients with SARS during that period of time.[5]

Roles of the Military Nurses

SongShan Armed Forces Hospital designated 188 nursing staff to care for patients with SARS. The nurses cared for 302 suspected patients with SARS. The process for isolating and caring for these patients relieved the epidemic situation of other hospitals and contributed significantly to the prevention and control of SARS for Taipei City. During the SARS outbreak, nurses fulfilled six different roles and functions in the SARS-dedicated hospitals: manager, caregiver, comfort provider, coordinator, advocate, and consultant.

Manager
The nurse managers were responsible for patient placement in the wards, ensuring infection control and disinfection measures were properly implemented. They also ensured that isolation interventions of the infectious patients were properly performed and that adequate supplies were available to maintain epidemic prevention strategies.

Caregiver
Usual nursing practices had to be altered because of the high infectious potential of SARS with close contact and within confined spaces. Nurses were required to wear full protection, which included a sealed protective gown, goggles, and N95 or P100 face masks and gloves whenever they were performing duties that required them to come in close contact with patients. Such duties covered a range of common nursing procedures, such as giving injections, administering other medications, turning patients, initiating nasogastric feedings, and providing assistance for toileting.

Comfort provider
Strict quarantine interventions were required for the patients with SARS. To avoid the risk of cross-infection, visiting hours were shortened and efforts were taken to minimize the frequency with which doors to the wards and rooms were opened. As a consequence, patients often spent less time with the nursing staff, friends, and relatives. The patients experienced a sense of enormous pressure and anxiety from the fear of the unknown associated with SARS, which resulted in many patients having issues with panic and insomnia. Some patients were even reluctant about cooperating

with the idea of isolation. Nurses, therefore, spent much time trying to understand the patients' emotional issues so they could provide them the comfort and support they needed. Often times, because of the limitations of isolation, this had to be accomplished over the patients' phone.

Coordinator
Nurses who were in the coordinator role communicated with patients and their families during the restructuring to a hospital dedicated exclusively to patients with SARS. The nurse coordinators also provided assistance during the transferring of inpatients so as not to interrupt their care. In the isolation wards, coordinators helped the nursing staff provide essential information to the mental health team who offered patients consultation, psychological counseling, appropriate information, necessary assistance, and relevant social resources. Coordinators contacted patients' family members and passed on messages related to their needs.

Infection control promotion
The nursing staff was also responsible for ensuring that medical staff members caring for patients on the wards were in full compliance with infection-control procedures, which included everyone from physicians and radiologists to the cleaning staff.

Consultant
The nursing staff served as consultants to educate patients about SARS, with the goal of reducing their fear of the disease. Education was tailored to the individual patient's needs. There were also many family members who felt anxious because they were not able to stay with patients on the wards. The nursing staff took a very proactive stance to try to reduce their anxiety by calling family members to keep them informed.

STRESS AND COPING OF UNIFORMED SERVICE NURSES ASSOCIATED WITH SEVERE ACUTE RESPIRATORY SYNDROME

The SARS epidemic rapidly spread within the medical institutions. There were incidents where medical and nursing staff died from the SARS infection, which had a profound effect on other front-line health care team members because they were very close to those who died. Deaths of staff and patients created an enormous amount of stress. Findings from a study by Yu and colleagues[12] showed that 50% of nursing staff felt a high degree of stress from working with patients during the SARS epidemic. The stress was experienced on many levels; there were many contributing factors. The nurses coped with this stress in various ways.

Stress
Staff members experienced physical stress as a result of caring for patients with SARS. As previously mentioned, the nursing staff was required to wear multiple layers of protective clothing when caring for patients. They were in the protective garb for long periods during their working hours. Air conditioners and electric fans, however, were prohibited on the wards housing the patients with SARS to reduce the spread of the virus, which made working conditions hot and humid. The combination of heavy protective clothing and the hot environmental conditions made it awkward to move, difficult to breathe, hard to hear, and left the nurses covered with sweat they were unable to wipe off. They also experienced urinary retention discomfort caused by limitations in going in and out of patients' rooms and not being able to easily remove the protective clothing.[13–15]

The caregivers also experienced significant psychological stressors. The SARS epidemic caused much fear within the Taiwanese society, but this was particularly felt among the nursing staff on several levels. They experienced fear of getting infected themselves. At the time, little was known about the SARS virus, including its lethality or how to best care for these patients. Nursing staff were very afraid of catching the SARS virus. Findings from studies done after the epidemic indicated the nursing staff believed their probability of getting infected by the SARS virus was between 53.85% to 71.9%.[16,17] The fear of being infected was not simply imagined because a member of the nursing staff in this hospital died from SARS.

The nurses also experienced fear of spreading the infection to their family members. Nursing staff were afraid if they became infected by SARS, they would pass on the virus to their family members. Based on findings from the study by Lin and colleagues,[18] 60% of the hospital staff, especially the nursing staff, thought people surrounding them did have a higher risk for becoming infected by SARS.

Fear of having to be isolated was another psychological stressor experienced by the nurses. There were two nurses from SongShan suspected of contracting the SARS virus; they were immediately admitted to isolation wards. These two nurses had been in contact with approximately 70 other nursing staff who were also placed on isolation. This frightened the rest of the nursing staff at the hospital. As a result, many of them prepared lists of things their family needed to do should they also be isolated. Some even prepared or passed on a will to their family members. According to a study by Chi and colleagues,[16] 52.35% of emergency health care staff feared that they would end up being isolated.

Another source of psychological stress surfaced from conflicts with professional ethics. At the beginning of the transfer of patients from Taipei hospitals to SongShan Armed Forces Hospital, nursing staff from both institutions found themselves at odds with the mission of containing the SARS epidemic and usual standards of nursing practice. Many usual patient care treatments were delayed or not done because of the environmental conditions (lack of air conditioning, discomfort, and protective clothing impediment); strict isolation measures; and the procedures put into place to handle the crisis. For example, nursing staff could not provide nebulizer inhalation treatments because of the restrictions in place to prevent the spread of SARS. Thus, there were limited treatment options when patients with SARS, who were too weak to cough and clear their airways, became short of breath from obstructed airways, which conflicted with what the nurses believed was ethical nursing practice. The nursing staff experienced a sense of severe powerlessness and guilt from these conflicts.[19-22]

There was also stress associated with caring for isolated and frightened patients. Patients with SARS were very frightened because of the strict quarantine interventions and because of the unknown characteristics of the virus itself. The patients exhibited symptoms of panic, emotional instability, and insomnia. Some even refused to cooperate with preventative isolation interventions, such as wearing facemasks. Some patients left the hospital without permission. The nursing staff was required to deal with these patients' fears and issues on a daily basis. The stress felt by the nursing staff exceeded the usual day-to-day stressors of nursing. There was a documented increase in the incidence of mental illness among the nursing staff involved with patients with SARS.[23]

Social stressors experienced by medical caregivers were especially heightened. The SARS outbreak was so terrifying that no one wanted family members to risk their lives caring for patients with SARS. Families also did not want to risk possible exposure to themselves by having a member working in the SARS hospitals. Consequently, some families refused to support the nurses' work. Not only did they try to stop the nurses from going to work but some even threatened the nurses with termination of their kin relationship. This added a social stress for the nurses.

Nurses caring for patients with SARS were also shunned by the public and people surrounding them. No restaurant would provide delivery service to the hospital. The nurses' family members were also shunned. For example, their spouses were forced to take temporary leave from work and their children were asked not to come to school during the SARS outbreak. These social phenomena gave the perception of discrediting the nursing profession. The military nursing staff at SongShan Armed Forces hospital had no choice but to go to work, and as a result they felt extremely frustrated and wronged.[13,14,21]

Similarly, the nursing staff was afraid of passing on the SARS virus to their family if they became infected. As a result, the nurses tried to avoid close contact with their family members and children as much as possible. They took the same precautions with their friends. These actions negatively affected their social lives and interpersonal relationships, leaving the nurses feeling isolated with little support.

Environmentally, because SARS was an emerging infectious disease with many unknowns, everyone involved was learning the latest preventative knowledge for the epidemic as they were experiencing it. Protective interventions and operating procedures were frequently changed during the course of the SARS epidemic adding further stress to an already stretched staff. Changes to government policies on SARS, such as sample collection, preventive measures, and medical procedures, occurred within short periods of time. Some of the logistical staff were afraid to enter the isolation wards during the outbreak, which meant normal repairs, such as replacement of broken equipment, was delayed or not done. This environmental stress added to the nurses' sense of helplessness and frustration.[21]

COPING

In 1984, Lazarus and Folkman[24] described emotion-oriented and problem-oriented coping behaviors. The emotion-oriented behaviors include adjusting one's coping mechanisms, such as seeking help to decrease reactions to added pressure. Problem-oriented behaviors include goal setting, gaining new knowledge about a situation, and learning new skills to directly decrease the pressure and therefore stress. The coping skills of the nursing staff at SongShan Armed Force Hospital are described based on this framework.

Emotion-oriented Behaviors

Maintaining a positive attitude
The nurses who worked during the SARS epidemic recognized their own professionalism during a time of stress. They felt proud of their abilities and their willingness to put aside some of their own fears to be on the front line of treating the patients with SARS and of preventing further illness and death.

Getting support from someone important
Support from family was valued most of all. Findings from a study conducted at Song-Shan Armed Forces Hospital showed that the support or non-support from family affected the staff members' willingness to care for patients with SARS.[25] Peer support among colleagues was also important to the nursing staff. Sharing emotional experiences with each other decreased their stress burden and helped them persevere during the epidemic.[13,20,21]

Hiding their feelings

During the epidemic, the nursing staff did not dare tell others about the kind of nursing work they were doing. They wanted to prevent fear and protect family members from the isolating actions of the general public. The results of a study by Lin and colleagues (2006) showed that 25% of health care staff avoided talking about the details of their work during the SARS outbreak.

Refraining from watching media coverage of the epidemic

SARS-related news adversely affected the emotions of the nursing staff. In addition to avoiding news and media reports, nursing staff tried to regulate their daily routine and lifestyle to also avoid contact and interaction with their neighbors and communities.[14]

Seeking spiritual support or accepting everything optimistically

The Taiwanese culture affected the nursing staff in that they believed caring for the patients with SARS was the right thing to do. The duty of nursing was to provide caring service for the patients. The nurses therefore believed the patients should not be abandoned no matter what happened. In performing this duty, they believed the end result would be good fortune and happiness.

Problem-oriented Behaviors

Seeking information

Nursing staff attended SARS training courses or they took the initiative to search for SARS-related information from the Internet. The hospital had an information board for SARS-related information and it held multidisciplinary discussion groups to ensure staff had accurate information about the virus, its characteristics, and symptoms. This sharing of information served to alleviate the stress levels of the staff.[13,15,20]

Using physical protection measures

The nurses used every standard infection-control measure available to prevent further spread of the infection. In addition to their protective clothing, they practiced diligent hand washing before, after, and between contacts with patients.

Balancing physiologic needs

Nurses minimized removing their protective clothing to attend to their own physiologic needs, which meant they decreased their water intake to avoid the need to use the bathroom. In addition, they consolidated tasks as much as possible to decrease energy expenditure and moving around while wearing the hot, heavy protective clothing in the hot, humid environment.

Maximizing health

The nurses realized they needed to ensure their own health so they attended to practices to increase their immunity. For example, they ensured they were eating a healthy diet and supplemented this with vitamins. In addition, they also tried to get as much sleep as possible and exercised daily.

Protecting family

The nursing staff believed they needed to keep their distance from family members and children when interacting with them. Many nurses simply temporarily stayed in the hostel that was provided by the hospital and settled family affairs either before moving to the hostel or via cell phone. This way they could care for the patients with SARS without having to worry about their family members getting the virus.

Adjusting daily activities

The nursing staff staying at the hostel also found ways to adjust their activities by such things as reading, watching television, and surfing the Internet. They used their cell phones for contact with their friends and family members. In this way, they were able to keep busy, yet still maintain their important social networks.

Evidence reflects that the better individuals adjust and optimize their own psychological and physical needs, the more effective they are during pressures like those accompanying an epidemic, such as SARS.[12] SARS-education training reduced the nursing staff's fear of becoming infected with SARS themselves or of infecting family members. This training also helped the staff reduce their negative feelings so they could engage in more healthy behaviors and maintain a positive attitude toward their patients' care.[26,27]

EVALUATION AND REVOLUTION AFTER SEVERE ACUTE RESPIRATORY SYNDROME ERA

The WHO removed Taiwan from its list of epidemic regions on July 5, 2003, which was only 4 months after Taiwan had its first case of SARS on March 14, 2003. There was still concern that with the arrival of fall and winter, SARS might make a comeback and overlap with the usual influenza season. There was fear that this potential overlap could again overwhelm the health care system. As a result, the Taiwanese government took the steps to prepare for this potential crisis.[1]

Fever screening was initiated. Because it was difficult to differentiate usual influenza and SARS, anyone with a fever was evaluated for SARS. Starting on August 19, 2003, any patients presenting to the emergency room with a fever was tested to rule out the SARS virus. Data as to virus types was used as a reference to making prevention and control policies.

An aggressive influenza vaccine program was started on September 15, 2003 to reduce the chance of pandemic influenza. All persons over the age of 65 years and all health care workers received free influenza vaccinations.

Patients with fevers were placed on isolation. The Centers for Disease Control set up a specified telephone line for fever consultation.[1] Patients with a fever were encouraged to wear masks and immediately isolate themselves at home for 3 days to avoid spreading their virus to other family members and the public.

The hospitals in Taiwan instituted fever surveillance systems for early detection of patients with fever and to take immediate precautionary interventions. Fever surveillance was also done in densely populated institutions, such as sanatoriums, preschools, and prisons. Information notification systems were implemented to track fever and disease patterns and to quickly notify the appropriate authorities of possible outbreaks of respiratory syndromes.

Border-control measures involving strict quarantine interventions were adopted on October 15, 2003 in an attempt to prevent another SARS or SARS-like epidemic from entering the country again. All incoming travelers who had fevers (body temperature over 38°C or 100.4°F) were immediately quarantined. This was reevaluated in November of the same year to determine if the practice should be continued.

Infection Control Teams were established to ensure patients did not develop nosocomial infection. The teams checked ventilation equipment, infection-control procedures, and participated in nosocomial prevention planning. The government performed 486 spot checks to ensure infection-control measures were properly implemented and any nosocomial infections appropriately treated.

The Taiwanese Center for Disease Control organized a National Infection Control network. The purpose of the network was to be ready to effectively use medical resources and the established institute infection-control mechanisms in the event of an epidemic. A total of 23 hospitals, distributed in different geographic areas throughout the country, were responsible for implementing the infection control policies.

On January 20, 2004, the Center for Disease Control disseminated the new version of the Communicable Disease Control Act. This Act defined infectious diseases and subdivided them into five categories. The categories were determined by degrees of risk, speed of transmission and mortality rates. SARS was placed in the first category, making it comparable to smallpox and plague. Other categories include specified infectious diseases, such as the avian flu and unknown emerging infectious.[28] The Act also spells out hospital related duties and implementation of control and preventive practices.[28,29] All the policies put into place after the SARS epidemic highlight the importance of hospital infection control they have permanently changed practices of health care providers. Some protective strategies include hand-washing habits, proper use of protective equipment, management of visitors and private duty nursing assistants, use of specific cleaning and disinfecting solutions, medical waste disposal, and safeguarding the environment.[1,30]

There were many lessons learned from the SARS epidemic in Taiwan. Because of the flexibility and sense of duty common among military personnel, SongShan Armed Forces General Hospital was able to quickly change its mission to provide first-line health care to patients with SARS during the epidemic. The value shown by the military nursing staff in the fight against SARS significantly impressed the citizens of the Taiwanese nation. The roles and mission that uniformed service nurses preformed was impressive. Their experiences and the hardships they endured provided valuable lessons for future health care crises. Although the impact of SARS greatly affected nursing staff physically and psychologically, it also provided them the opportunity to reflect on issues related to the nursing profession. With regard to nursing practice, nurses should have an increased awareness of emerging infectious diseases. Stress-management methods can help them deal with some of the difficulties experienced during public health crises. The authors think these lessons can only strengthen the dignity of the profession and enhance nurses' abilities for future emergent events.[20] The SARS epidemic in Taiwan ushered in a new era for infectious-disease treatment and prevention in epidemic control and the development of specific management strategies.

REFERENCES

1. Center for Disease Control. SARS control key record in Taiwan. Taiwan: Taipei Center for Disease Control, Department of Health; 2004.
2. World Health Organization. Severe acute respiratory syndrome SARS -multi-country outbreak-Update 49 7 May 2007. Available at: http//www.who.int/csr/don/2003_05_07a/en. Accessed April 22, 2009.
3. Huang HH, Yen DH, Kao WF, et al. Declining emergency department visits and costs during the severe acute respiratory syndrome SARS outbreak. J Formos Med Assoc 2006;105(1):31–7.
4. Chen R, Chou KR, Huang YJ, et al. Effect of a SARS prevention program in Taiwan on nursing staff's anxiety, depression and sleep quality: a longitudinal survey. Int J Nurs Stud 2006;43:215–25.
5. The Ministry of National Defense. The national troops prevent and control SARS on-the-spot report. Taipei (Taiwan): The Ministry of National Defense; 2003.

6. Chen SQ, Tu WS. SARS epidemic situation to tourism and shipping industry influence. National Policy Forum; 2003. p. 49–60.
7. Wei D. To SARS event the impact and countermeasure of Taiwan economy. National Policy Forum; 2003. p. 19–30.
8. Chen SC, Jo YJ, Lin JR, et al. The analysis of economic loss and responsible expedients during severe acute respiratory syndrome (SARS) for hospitality in Taiwan. Review of Tourism and Hospitality 2007;1(1):105–29.
9. Lin MX, Tseng HD. The discussion for special budgeting and implementing of central government SARS preventing and controlling strategy. Finance Officer Monthly Publication 2006;608:11–5.
10. Chiu RN, Che YR. The crisis management strategy of heavy epidemic crisis in central government-experiences of SARS in M.O.C. Community Dev J 2003; 104:4–11.
11. Center for Disease Control. Memoir of Severe Acute Respiratory Syndrome Control in Taiwan. Taiwan: Taipei Center for Disease Control, Department of Health; 2003.
12. Yu WC, Li SH, Yuan SC, et al. Job stress and coping in emergency room nurses confronting severe acute respiratory syndrome crisis. Chung Shan Medical Journal 2007;18(1):25–41.
13. Guo JN, Lee BE, Lee CX. Work-related stress and coping behaviors during SARS outbreak period among emergency nurses in Taiwan. Chang Gung Nursing 2005; 16(2):139–51.
14. Chen SL, Huang YP, Tsai SF, et al. Nursing experiences and coping behaviors of caring for a child with suspected SARS a focus group approach. Chang Gung Nursing 2005;16(3):275–87.
15. Pan HH, Chiu CK, Chiu CP. Stress and coping behaviors of nurses caring for patients with SARS: an exploratory descriptive study. Journal of Taiwan Nephrology Nursing Association 2003;2(2):120–8.
16. Chi HT, Liao CC, Hu WH, et al. Concepts and attitudes toward SARS ordinary Taiwanese versus medical staff. Journal of Taiwan Emergency Medical 2003; 6(1):1–12.
17. Shiao JS, Koh D, Lo LH, et al. Factors predicting nurse' consideration of leaving their job during the SARS outbreak. Nurs Ethics 2007;14(1):5–17.
18. Lin YC, Guo YL, Lo LH, et al. Perception of risk and preventive measures among health care workers after the SARS outbreak in Taiwan. Chinese Journal of Occupational Medicine 2006;13(1):39–46.
19. Chen LL, Fang JT. Severe Acute Respiratory Syndrome Diagnosis and Management. Journal of Taiwan Nephrology Nursing Association 2003;2(2):90–7.
20. Hung HC, Weng LC, Fang CY. Stresses and adjustment behaviors of surgical nurses caring for SARS patients. Evid Based Nurs 2005;1(1):45–51.
21. Pan SM, Feng MC, Wu MH, et al. Voices from the frontline: nurses' impact and coping during the 2003 SARS outbreak in Southern Taiwan. Evid Based Nurs 2005;1(2):149–56.
22. Chiang SS, Chen MB, Su YL. Ethical dilemmas in caring for patients with SARS. The Journal of Nursing 2006;53(5):28–34.
23. Chen QZ, Guo QZ, Lee MB. Effect of the severe acute respiratory syndrome epidemic on psychiatric morbidity of medical personnel. Taipei City Medical Journal 2004;1(1):75–80.
24. Lazarus RS, Folkman S. Stress appraisal and coping. New York: Springer; 1984.
25. Chen TJ, Lin MH, Chou LF, et al. Hospice utilization during the SARS outbreak in Taiwan. BMC Health Serv Res 2006;6:94–100.

26. Su TP, Lien TC, Yang CY, et al. Prevalence of psychiatric morbidity and psychological adaptation of the nurses in a structured SARS caring unit during outbreak a prospective and periodic assessment study in Taiwan. J Psychiatr Res 2007; 41(1–2):119–30.

27. Tzeng HM. Nurses' professional care obligation and their attitudes towards SARS infection control measures in Taiwan during and after the 2003 epidemic. Nurs Ethics 2004;113:277–89.

28. Center for Disease Control. Communicable Disease Control Act 2004b. Available at: http//www.cdc.gov.tw/public/Data/911314141071.doc. Accessed July 18, 2009.

29. Chu DC, Hu BS, Huang YN, et al. The amended infectious disease law and its impacts on hospital management. Taipei City Medical Journal 2005;23:232–9.

30. Chen YY. Infection control after the outbreak of severe acute respiratory syndrome. VGH Nursing 2003;20(4):378–86.

Hard Labor: The Personal Experiences of Two Obstetric Nurses in Balad, Iraq

Katrina Poole, RNC, BSN, MA[a],*, Angela Lacek, RN, BSN, MSHS[b]

KEYWORDS
- Obstetric nurses • War • Nursing roles • Deployment

Nurses are inherently linked to care of injured soldiers on battlefields worldwide. During wartime assignments, nurses may be required to care for patients whose needs are outside their usual clinical expertise. A great deal of literature describes eyewitness accounts and provides summaries of the roles nurses have fulfilled and their perceptions of nursing during war. A common theme throughout these writings is that nurses expressed a lack of preparation for what they would do and what they would find in the battlefield hospitals.[1–5] Griffiths and Jasper[6] described military nurses as having dual identities: that of a traditional professional nurse, caring for ill patients in many settings, and that of being a "soldier," willing to go where needed, but also requiring training and preparation for many new and different roles.

In Iraq and Afghanistan, nurses are at the core of the health care provided to service members and civilians who incur war injuries. In this article, two Air Force obstetric nurses who deployed to Balad, Iraq describe their personal experiences and explore the challenges they faced while practicing outside their specialty of obstetric nursing. One nurse worked as a medical-surgical nurse and the other as an emergency room (ER) nurse. Although their experiences were mentally and physically exhausting, both found them to be extremely rewarding.

NURSE 1: AN OBSTETRIC NURSE... IN BALAD

After 14 years as an Air Force nurse, I had never had the opportunity to deploy to either a war zone or on a humanitarian mission. Opportunity may seem like a strange choice

The opinions or assertions contained herein are solely the views of the authors and should not be construed as official or reflecting the views of the United States Air Force, the Department of Defense or United States Government.

[a] Perinatal Unit, Elmendorf Air Force Base Hospital, Elmendorf Air Force Base, 5955 Zeamer Avenue EAFB, AK 99506, USA

[b] Family Medicine, 87th Medical Group, McGuire Air Force Base, NJ 08641, USA

* Corresponding author.
E-mail address: katrina.poole@elmendorf.af.mil

of words; however, for most military nurses, this is exactly how deployment is viewed. As military nurses, we begin training for deployment shortly after becoming members of the nurse corps. In May 2006, while stationed at Wilford Hall Medical Center in San Antonio, Texas, I was told I would deploy in support of Operation Iraqi Freedom. As I scanned the tasking letter, a range of emotions overcame me: fear, excitement, and apprehension. I had so many questions. I had specialized in obstetric (OB) nursing and I knew there were no "OB units" in Balad. What would I do there? My situation had an added twist because I had been in administrative positions for the last 7 years! I was suddenly overwhelmed by fear… fear of failure, fear of the unknown and fear of those around me finding out about my fear! Like most nurses, failure is never an option, but I was not sure how to overcome my extreme knowledge deficit in such a short time.

I soon discovered that nurses who were not intensive care or ER nurses were placed on the medical-surgical ward in a field hospital. I had not worked with medical-surgical patients in 10 years; however, I was suddenly very thankful for having had that experience. I was quite nervous at the thought of caring for anyone other than obstetric patients. I have always supported the idea that novice nurses should have at least 1 year of medical-surgical nursing before specializing. My experience in Balad was confirmation of that belief.

Once I absorbed the reality of being expected to work outside my comfort zone, I had to begin the monumental task of preparing to leave. When I deployed to Balad, a deployment cycle (the number of days a service member is deployed) was 120 days for Air Force nurses, which seemed like an eternity. Shortly after receiving official notification of my deployment, I was bombarded with a multitude of tasks, briefings, and trainings. These events had to be accomplished within a specific timeframe. I was trained on the use of weapons, such as an M-9 handgun. I attended field training, which taught me about living in desert conditions and how to recognize and protect myself from poisonous snakes and spiders. During chemical warfare training, I was taught how to properly wear a gas mask and a chemical protective suit. Time became a priceless commodity during the preparation phase of deployment, so I scrutinized every moment of my day. The demands of my normal duty schedule, preparations for deployment, and my family needs became overwhelming. Much had to be done to prepare my family for my absence; my husband and two teenage daughters were quite nervous that I would be traveling into a warzone.

Several classes were available to help me prepare for the type of patients that I would encounter during deployment. The Trauma Nurse Course and Burn Course at Brooke Army Medical Center were excellent resources that provided realistic, hands-on training. Several other courses were available, but time constraints prevented me from taking them all. I had to accept that I might not know everything about my patients and equipment before leaving.

Back to the Bedside

After the training and checklist were completed, I said goodbye to my family and friends. I was prepared to leave San Antonio. The day of departure could not have been more fitting for me and the other OB nurse; it was Labor Day! Retrospectively, I really wish someone had told me to travel a lot lighter! I had 4 duffle bags, each weighing approximately 15 to 20 lb. Thankfully, people helped me carry some of my bags.

The flight to Balad included several stops; altogether, the trip was 96 hours. Because of a scheduling error, when we arrived at our initial stop there was no designated place for us to sleep. We slept in the library, on benches, chairs, or wherever we could find a soft spot. Additionally, we were grounded at our initial stop for a few days, because of mechanical problems with the plane, further delaying our arrival into Balad. The delay was painful. On numerous occasions we were told our plane was ready, but after we had gathered our belongings, we were told the wait would continue. To make things worse, a great deal of our waiting was done outside in grueling heat. We arrived in Balad thoroughly exhausted.

On arrival in Balad, my first priority was a hot shower and a good night's sleep. However, the shower and sleep were preempted by our orientation. We were bussed to a briefing room on base and given instructions on base rules and regulations. After the orientation, we were taken to get our bags. We were then sent to the housing office where we waited in line for hours to be given our rooms. Finally, I received the key to my room and dragged my four bags with me. Shortly after getting our bags into our rooms, we were told to report to the hospital for a tour and briefing. We had just traveled thousands of miles. We were dirty, exhausted, and terribly hungry. But we gathered our wits, found the hospital, and waited patiently in the cafeteria where the hospital commander welcomed us.

After the commander's briefing, I got a quick glimpse of the various types of patients for whom I would be caring. What little confidence I may have acquired escaped me. I saw individuals with extensive abdominal wounds, double amputations, and various facial traumas. As an OB nurse, I was beginning to realize just how far out of my comfort zone I would be in caring for these patients. Next, we were gathered and told by our flight commander what shift we would be working, which had obviously been decided before we arrived. I was on night shift. Others told me that night shift was good because of the time difference. Balad is 9 hours ahead of San Antonio, so being on night shift would be like being on day shift back home.

We were expected to shadow our assigned preceptors for the remainder of their shift, At this point I only had two things on my mind: food and sleep. We were told we would only have 2 days of overlap/orientation to learn our new jobs. This announcement met with much grumbling and protesting, but to no avail! Approximately 5 hours after initially arriving in Balad, we were released to eat and get a few hours of rest. I slept for approximately 4 hours before returning for a 12-hour shift.

I had many questions, and tried to carve out as much time with my preceptor as I could. It was not until later that we learned the rationale for the hasty release of our predecessors: there was not enough housing to accommodate both the departing and arriving personnel on the base for an extended amount of time. In addition, it placed extra demands on food services. These issues are just some that you do not consider when you are not involved with the logistical planning of changing out an entire hospital staff all at once. Having that piece of the puzzle made things much easier to understand.

My first night on duty was overwhelming. After not caring for patients in approximately 10 years, I had eight patients who had an assortment of drains, dressing changes, and tracheostomy care. In addition to the patient load, we received a "Balad welcome" (our first mortar attack), and spent approximately 20 minutes under our patients' cots after an alarm red, which is signified by sirens and a loud booming voice on the Public Address (PA) system that can be heard over the entire base saying… "ALARM RED! ALARM RED!" We called it the *giant voice*. When I heard the giant voice I knew we had been attacked and had to put on what was known as my *battle rattle*: my helmet and flack vest. I then had to find a safe place to take cover, which sometimes was under my patient's cot!

As days passed, I became more familiar with my environment. It was dirty, noisy, and smelly. Often, patients would cry out for pain medications and the television played constantly, which quickly became a nuisance to me. The unit reeked of unwashed bodies and bad breath. The helicopter made frequent landings, bringing in dust and more wounded. The noise and dust with each landing was incredible. I quickly learned what was most important to the patients in my care; their priorities were pain control, knowing they were safe, and having someone listen to their stories. They were so grateful for the care they received.

Several medical-surgical nurses on my shift were readily available to answer any questions I had regarding patient care. It was imperative that each nurse had the skills to properly care for 6 to 7 patients each night. What you did not learn before arriving, you quickly picked up through on-the-job training from a skilled nurse. Despite the less-than-desirable conditions, the patients received state-of-the-art care, in the middle of the desert, in a tent hospital! Before I knew it, I had forgotten that I was an OB nurse. I was managing chest tubes, patients recovering from orthopedic surgery, and patients who had numerous traumatic injuries. The versatility of the military nurse came to the foreground and I no longer felt so far out of my comfort zone.

Although most of my patients were adult men, we occasionally received pediatric patients who were injured by suicide bombers or improvised explosive devices. Some were burned by gas heaters used to warm the Iraqi homes during the cold winter months. In addition to the normal issues pediatric patients have, such as fear and distrust when in a hospital setting, the language barrier and cultural issues magnified those challenges. The compassion I had for the children was difficult to convey through a translator. Every effort was made to put nurses with pediatric experience with those patients. However, that was not always possible, so we all had to learn to be pediatric nurses, which was another test that showed our versatility. Regardless of our nursing background, we all came prepared to learn skills outside our specialty, and we did.

Despite heroic efforts, we were not able to save everyone. Some patients were so severely injured that our major intervention was to provide comfort. I became skilled at postmortem care. No matter the age or nationality of the deceased, preparing a body for the morgue was never easy, and is something obstetric nurses rarely must do. I found this part of my job really difficult. I never became desensitized or unmoved by the loss of life, no matter how many times it happened. Occasionally we lost children, sometimes entire families, and our soldiers.

In addition to my duties as a staff nurse on a ward, I was a night supervisor. The role of a nursing supervisor is to help with patient placement within the field hospital, ensuring each patient has access to the care needed. I made certain a bed was available in the intensive care unit or the ward when the patient was ready to be moved from the ER after triage and stabilization.

The nursing supervisor also responds to trauma calls, exposing me to some of the most disturbing aspects of my deployment. Trauma patients generally arrived at the hospital by helicopter, and the ER staff would receive an alert before it arrived. Seeing trauma patients fresh from the field with no limbs, open abdominal wounds, and gaping head wounds was something I was not prepared for; getting used to this took some time. During trauma calls there is no such thing as an obstetric nurse or a medical-surgical nurse. No one knows who you are or what your background is; you learn to use the skills you acquired on the job, and that is how you gain respect. Trauma calls in the ER truly put it all together. All of the training comes to the forefront, and everyone has a role. I saw several lives lost and many more saved.

NURSE 2: OBSTETRIC NURSE TO EMERGENCY ROOM NURSE, MY EXPERIENCE IN BALAD

The ER is probably one of the most challenging places to work in the field hospital. I was deployed to Balad to work in the ER, and I returned from Iraq as a much different person. I came home a much better nurse. I now know that as an Air Force Officer I have the skills I need to survive and thrive in any environment. I could not have imagined any of this when I was commissioned in the United States Air Force in December of 2003.

I wanted to go into the Air Force since graduating from nursing school in 1995, but having young children kept me from entering the service. My husband, also an Air Force Officer, feared the possibility of us both needing to deploy at the same time and having nobody to watch our children. In 2003, our children were 12, 8, and 6 years of age, all in school, and old enough to understand our service and potential sacrifice should we be called away. I talked in depth to other military nurses about their experiences. Most of them loved their military service and the associated opportunities. After much soul searching and family discussion, we decided it was the right decision—I was joining the Air Force.

My first duty assignment was Royal Air Force Base, Lakenheath, England. After spending 3 years assigned in England, my next assignment was to the Birthing Center at Wilford Hall Medical Center (WHMC) at Lackland Air Force Base in San Antonio, Texas. I was surprised to learn that two of the OB nurses stationed at Wilford Hall were deployed to Iraq. I talked to my supervisor, who informed me that our unit deployed OB nurses regularly. In fact, my supervisor was deploying in September 2006. When I told my husband that my supervisor was scheduled to deploy, he shrugged it off. After all, though he had deployed, he had never been to Iraq, so what were the chances that I would go first? He had more of a combat mission in the Air Force, being a Security Forces Officer. Certainly, OB nurses were not needed in a war zone, so he never really thought I would be sent to Iraq. The possibility that I might deploy was always in the back of my mind. However, I rationalized I was a labor and delivery nurse—not a combat medic—and I was not going to a war zone.

Nevertheless, two or three nurses from our unit deployed to Iraq every cycle. I attended Medical Unit Readiness Training, learning and performing various combat skills and scenarios in full chemical gear. Chemical gear is a charcoal lined suit, rubber gloves, rubber boots, and a gas mask. I learned about the potential deployment hazards and attended weapons training. It all seemed a little far-fetched to me; I would tell my husband about it when I got home and we would laugh about how silly it seemed that a nurse—an OB nurse at that—would have to have this training. In November 2006, I was told that I would deploy to the Air Force hospital in Balad, Iraq. My whole family was in a bit of shock. It was exciting and scary at the same time and I knew my life would never be the same.

I talked with many OB nurses who had already deployed; they all told me it was the best experience of their professional career. A friend and coworker talked in depth about working on the intensive care ward in Balad. She told me stories that were endearing, heart wrenching, and sometimes funny. At times I wanted to cry, and at others I laughed so hard I did cry—for her. The hardest part of her deployment seemed to be leaving her family, and I knew I would have that same problem. But she constantly assured me that the experience was worth having, and that my training as an OB nurse would get me through, as it did her.

Two weeks before I left for Iraq, I received an email entitled "Welcome to the ER." Certainly, that was a mistake, because I was going to work on the intensive care ward, like every other OB nurse who had deployed to Balad from Lackland Air Force Base, and where my supervisor was currently working. I sent my supervisor an email so I could clear up the misunderstanding, and was a little shocked at her reply. Apparently, there was a shortage of ER nurses, and the hospital leadership at WHMC and the Air Force Theater Hospital (AFTH) decided I would be great in that role. I was extremely nervous, but my supervisor assured me that I would do a great job and should not worry. I felt honored my leaders believed I would do well, but also apprehensive. My supervisor encouraged me to work a few days in the WHMC ER to get some experience, so I did. For 1 day. No traumas occurred. Nothing at all prepared me for what I would experience during my deployment.

I left for Iraq on January 9, 2007. What a sad day at my house. When I came out of the bedroom that morning, my 15-year-old son and our 17-year-old exchange student were at the kitchen table talking quietly. When I walked in, my son looked at me with sad, tearful eyes, and our exchange student burst into a full-fledged sob. I hugged both kids, trying to reassure them they would be fine with dad and that I would be safe. The other two kids came downstairs, both looking sad, but holding up better than the teenagers.

I walked my 10-year-old son, our youngest, to the school bus stop and we talked a little bit about what I would be doing and when I would be home. He promised me he would help daddy at the house and he would take care of our dog. As the school bus pulled up, I thought my heart would break. I would not see my baby again for quite some time and I did not know how I would get through. He was such a big boy, and he assured me that he would be fine. I hugged and kissed him, and then I stood and waved at him until the bus turned and was out of sight. I was a wreck, and I had not even left the house yet!

I went inside where my 12-year-old daughter was getting ready to leave for school. Always the hardheaded, strong-willed child, she gave me a quick hug, told me not to worry, and asked why everyone was crying. She shrugged off her worries, grabbed her bag, and made a pouty face at her brother for crying (that's my tough girl!). She assured me that she would miss me, she just was not crying because she is "not the emotional type." With that, she was out the front door. My husband gave me a big hug and made sure I knew my daughter loved me, but she was dealing with my leaving in her own way, I knew he was right.

The older two teenagers were still sitting at the table crying, and informed my husband they would not be attending school that day. We nodded, understanding they needed time to grieve my absence, even though it was only for a few months. Although none of us openly said it, we all knew I was going to a dangerous place, and there was a small possibility that I would not return.

My husband and I drove quietly to the hospital, where I was scheduled to meet with my deployment team—a group of approximately 80 Air Force medics (doctors, nurses, and technicians). He and I said goodbye, and as we were hugging I realized that all of the times he deployed to various locations, I never knew how difficult it was for him to leave his family behind. I just took it for granted that he loved his job, and leaving us was a small sacrifice. How naïve I had been. My husband was such a good man, and at that moment I realized all he had sacrificed for the betterment of our family. I knew that my kids would be in good hands with their daddy, and that they would take care of each other.

After he left, I went into the hospital auditorium to begin my life-changing journey. I sat there crying and I felt silly, but I do not think there were many dry eyes in the room. I took pictures on the bus and in the deployment processing center, not realizing the future I would share with these people who I barely knew at this point. Four months later, when I looked back at those pictures, the faces meant so much more to me than they did that day.

We made seven stops before arriving in Balad. I rested some, cried a lot, but mainly just worried about what the next 4 months would bring. One of our stops lasted for 2 days. We arrived in Balad, Iraq on January, 13th. I was surprised to realize Iraq was not hot; in fact, the weather was a lot like San Antonio. It had recently rained in Balad, and mud was everywhere.

We were bused to our housing area, and while awaiting our room assignments, I heard an explosion and gunfire. The civilian contractor giving us our housing briefing did not miss a beat, shrugged off the explosion, and continued. I was not sure what had just happened, but my heart was racing a mile a minute! Once I received my room key, I started dragging my bags toward my room. I had been warned to travel light, and had only two bags, but the mud was so thick and my bags so heavy that I did not know how I was going to get there. I looked around, and the reality hit me. I was in Iraq, I was alone, and I was scared to death. I was choking back tears wondering how in the hell I was going to get to my room, when two medics, who I would later work with, came to my rescue. They helped me get my bags to my room and told me when and where everyone was meeting up for dinner. I was so grateful!

After dinner, I unpacked and decided to take a shower. We lived in small trailers, and the nearest Cadillac (slang for bathrooms that were not port-a-potties), was a few city blocks away. As I was doing my best to navigate through the puddle, I lost my shoe. The mud sucked it right off my foot! Ewe! Outside, it was dark, scary, quiet, and dirty! I somehow made it through the first night alone and scared to death. I was not able to call home, and I was so sad—I missed my family so much!

The next day, we met at the hospital dining facility at 7 AM to start work. As I was walking through the tent hospital I saw my supervisor from WHMC; I was so happy! But she had all of her bags packed and with her; she was leaving that day. She gave me a quick hug, assured me that I would do a great job, and then she was gone. I was alone again, waiting for someone to tell me what the heck I was doing.

A nurse from the ER came to get me, telling me how glad he was that I arrived so he could leave that day. I wondered if he was joking, because surely they would not let the person I was replacing leave until I knew what I was doing. He gave me a quick tour of the hospital, introduced me to the outgoing nurse manager, and he was gone. I never saw him again. The outgoing nurse manager looked at me very suspiciously. He sipped on his coffee and eyed me. I suspect he was wondering if I would be able to handle being an ER nurse. I wondered that too. The nurse manager told me I could make some phone calls or go back to my trailer for a few hours, because my shift did not start until noon. I would be working noon-to-moon (12 PM–12 AM) because that would ensure I would never have to staff the ER without a qualified ER nurse being present. I was extremely grateful for that, and knew that he was still looking at me, wondering if I would sink or swim.

I called home, talked to my husband, and told him how scared I was. As always, he reassured me that I would be fine. He has always been my biggest fan—he has more faith in me and my abilities than I will ever have. Talking to him made me feel so much better, but also made me realize how homesick I was. I already missed my family and I had only been gone for 6 days, and I had 114 to go.

When I arrived back in the ER that afternoon, I met the incoming nurse manager. She assured me that I would do fine and told me if I had any questions, she would help me. Around 2 PM, we had our first real patients. My patient was a 3-year-old girl who had been shot in the head by a sniper. I helped the surgeon remove the dressing from her head and a big piece of her skull was missing. I was literally holding this poor baby's brain in my hand. We performed a CT scan, and found that, just as we suspected, her wounds were fatal. The entire time we were working on her, her father sat on a bench at the end of a trauma bay watching.

Once the physician determined we could not save her, we started providing comfort measures. We put up privacy curtains out of respect, and I cleaned her little body the best I could. The interpreter came to talk to the father, who just shook his head but did not come to his daughter's side, even when offered. After she passed away, we wheeled her body to the morgue, which was on the other side of the bench where her father was sitting. He had tears in his eyes, but aside from that I could see no emotion. He reached up and patted his daughter's body as we passed by, then left the ER. Approximately 30 minutes later, after he completed all the paperwork, he came back to get her, and very stoically carried her little body out of the ER. I was mortified. How could any parent be so devoid of emotion after losing a child? I could not comprehend it, and it made me simultaneously miss my kids and grieve for that little girl.

Even though I was on an emotional rollercoaster, I felt pretty good about my nursing performance so far. OB nurse or not, I could do this. I was working with three other nurses, and we were helping each other and things were going great. So far, we had received patients one or two at a time throughout the day, and the ER doctors and surgeons were right by our sides. But I had no idea what the night would bring.

Every night, the AFTH would get American patients from all over Iraq en route to Germany. Most of our patients came from an Army hospital in Baghdad. A lot of combat action occurred in the early months of 2007, and I was about to see firsthand the devastation of war. At approximately 6 PM the night nurses arrived. I met another ER nurse from WHMC that night. She was the person I spent the most time with over the next 4 months, and ironically she lived only approximately 5 miles from me in San Antonio.

At about 10 PM that night, we started receiving our aeromedical evacuation patients. It was overwhelming. They just kept coming in wave after wave of helicopter traffic. I really do not know how many, but there were a lot of helicopters. Some service members we triaged went straight to the operating room for surgery. Some needed blood transfusions, some pain medicine. Some were experiencing combat stress and needed a shoulder to cry on. All of them needed to go home, and our job was to make sure they got there.

At midnight, it was time for me to leave. The events of the day weighed heavily on my shoulders (or maybe that was the 50 lb that I was carrying in flack vest, helmet, and backpack). All I could think of was the numerous traumatic injuries throughout the day that we could not save. Either way, it was incredibly dark, quiet, and eerie. I walked as fast as I could on the desolate base, wondering if I was going to get shot, mugged, or mortared. I got to my room, trying to be quiet and not wake my roommate, who worked the dayshift. I changed and went to bed. I was too scared to walk to the showers—that would have to wait until morning. I looked at the pictures of my family and cried myself to sleep. I really felt out of my element, wondered how I had gotten here, and what was ahead of me.

The next day, I was back in the ER at noon. I felt better than the night before but was still apprehensive about the day ahead. I had written down all of the medications from the previous day that I did not know and looked up all of them. We did not have barcode medication administration support, but we did have a very good reference library in the hospital. I reviewed all of the medications, diagnoses, policies, and procedures that I could find. For 2 weeks, I read everything I could find, and if I could not find it, I asked the other nurses and doctors. On some level, I felt foolish because I had been a nurse much longer than some of the people I was asking for help, but I reassured myself that if they were in my world (OB), they would need me in the same way.

On the rare occasion that we got a pregnant patient or an infant, I was in my element. These were all "my patients," and even the ER doctors referred to me for their care. However, these patients were few and far between. Most of our patients during the day were Iraqi civilians, and many were children. We received the air evacuation patients every night. The ER crew was becoming a team, and I was a part of that team, even as an OB nurse.

At the hospital, we were usually too busy to think about what we were doing. We were caring for people with horrific injuries. But my first week in Balad, I cried myself to sleep every night. I tried to keep a journal of my experiences, but found it too painful. As I wrote, I would cry, and I hated reliving those experiences. Eventually, I stopped writing in my journal.

One day at work, one of the enlisted medics commented that he had never seen me cry. I looked at him in a puzzled way, and he told me that I looked "like a cry baby," but he never saw that side of me. I realized he was right; I had never cried at work, only in my room at night, and I stopped doing that after the first week. I was becoming emotionally detached from everything, even the patients that I took care of...even my family. My husband commented on it more than once when we talked on the phone. I did let my emotional wall down a few times, but very little.

One night, we received a group of patients injured in a mortar attack on their house. Most were children, and I was caring for a 7-year-old girl. Her mother was with her, uninjured and sitting on the bench. Despite all of our efforts to save her life, the little girl did not survive. I called for the interpreter, and had him explain to the mother what happened. She appeared extremely distraught, letting out the most gut-wrenching cry I had heard in Iraq. She embraced me and cried, all while repeating the same phrase over and over. As a mother myself, I felt an emotional connection to this woman. Even though we were from two different worlds, I felt we had a kinship as mothers—I felt her pain. I cried with her, returned her embrace, and let her grieve. I think I was grieving in my own way, too.

When it was over and the mother left with her little girl's body, I asked the interpreter what she was saying, because she kept repeating the same phrase over and over. He did not directly answer my question, just replied that she was very upset. I asked him to tell me what she was saying, and again he gave me an indirect answer. I then told him not to hide anything or try to spare my feelings, and I had to know what she kept repeating in her grief over her daughter's death. Very reluctantly, he told me the mother was afraid to tell her husband the daughter had died for fear he would kill her, and she kept repeating over and over for him to have pity on her and not beat her for their daughter's death. I felt so foolish. I really thought she was grieving the loss of her daughter, the way I would grieve the loss of one of my children. But instead she was fearful for her own life. I was incredibly angry, and I silently vowed that I would never let down my emotional guard again.

Looking back, I think guarding my emotions was how I protected myself from the harsh realities I faced every day. Maybe it was my desire to be as good an ER nurse as I am an OB nurse, and I poured myself into learning and getting better at my job. I am not really sure. Even today, I know I am not the same person emotionally that I was when I arrived in Iraq. That experience took a toll on my emotions.

Other days were also emotionally draining. I was devastated when the first American service member I cared for died. He had a fatal gunshot wound to his head. He was very young, 19 or 20 years old, and after the physician removed him from life support,

I held his hand as he passed away. I know he did not know I was there, but all I could think about was his family—his mother especially—and the fact they would appreciate knowing that I stayed with him while he died.

Another especially hard loss was a service member who came in after being trapped in his vehicle in a roadside bomb explosion. He had burns on 90% of his body, but he was awake and talking when he arrived in the ER. He told me his name and I assured him we would take good care of him. I managed to start an intravenous line, gave him some pain medication, and helped quickly sedate and get him intubated. The whole ER team was vigorously working to save his life when the surgeon entered the trauma bay. He took one look at his injuries and told us to stop resuscitative measures because his injuries were nonsurvivable. Looking back, I knew he was right, but at that time I could not get past the fact that 10 minutes earlier this service member and I were talking. That was one of my darker days in Iraq—one that still haunts me—but again I did not cry.

I did write my most memorable patients' names in my journal so I would never forget their sacrifices for this country and the Iraqi people. I often wonder if I should contact their family members and let them know that their loved one was not alone at the end, but I honestly do not know if this would be the right thing. Sometimes I think it would help my grief, but I do not know if it would help the families, and the last thing I want to do is cause them more pain.

After a couple of months, I think I resembled an ER nurse. One slow night, another nurse and I were talking and the ER doctors and technicians were playing foosball in the trauma bay (can you believe someone sent us a foosball table?). One of our technicians came into the ER and said a patient was in the parking lot. We went outside to see if the patient needed help, and when I saw the patient's arm flop out the door of the vehicle he was in, I knew we were in trouble. The other nurse went to the car, and I ran inside to get a stretcher. I yelled for help, and when we returned with the patient, we all got to work. The patient was in cardiac arrest and I directed the resuscitative efforts. The patient was a Turkish contractor and his friends had no idea how long he had been down before they found him. He was cold to the touch and his pupils were fixed and dilated on arrival. We briefly got a pulse but nothing sustainable. Even though we were unable to save his life, I felt so good knowing that I truly tried and was not scared or apprehensive to treat him. Although we worked for 45 minutes to save his life, the effort was futile. My friend says that was the day I became an ER nurse.

The last few weeks of my time in Iraq flew by. We were scheduled to leave around the middle of May, and Nurses Week was the 2nd week of May. Yes, even in Iraq Nurses Week is recognized. The hospital leaders planned a dinner and awards ceremony in honor of our hard work during our stay there.

The commander presented awards to the nurses in each area. It was nice to see nurses rewarded for their hard work and dedication. When the ER nurse award was given, the nurse manager talked about what a great leader our number one nurse was, always teaching everyone a new skill and helping coworkers, never afraid to get dirty or ask for help if needed. It was so nice, and I was truly thinking that she was describing my friend. To my great surprise, my name was announced as the number one ER nurse; I was so humbled and honored. When I arrived in Balad, never in a million years did I think I would leave feeling like an ER nurse, nor could I imagine receiving such a great honor from my coworkers and leaders. I have earned many awards during my time in the military, but none have meant as much to me as this award. I worked hard at my job every day, and I never forgot that even though I was out of my element, these patients counted on me for their lives and I could not let them down. I tried to care for each one of them as if they were my family members—my husband, my children. I knew I could not live with myself if I did not give 100% every day, and that is exactly what I did.

As I write this, it has been almost 2 years to the day since I returned home from Iraq. Some aspects of my journey are in my head as if they happened yesterday, and others are fading quickly. The words I have written are just a small glimpse of my deployment experiences. I cared for young American service men and women who experienced horrors beyond my imagination. I cared for people who lived lives I cannot even comprehend.

I hope that the young children of Iraq whose lives have been devastated by war will remember the American service members as kind people who helped save their lives. I hope the service members who were severely injured will know their sacrifices did not go unnoticed, and that we worked as hard to preserve their lives as they worked at preserving our freedom. I would like the parents and spouses who lost family members under my watch to know I stayed with their loved ones until the end, holding their hand and providing comfort during their darkest hour. I hope that my children understand the time they lost with their mother was worth the sacrifice. I know that my husband understands this because he lived it also.

I returned from Iraq as a much different person from when I left. I came home to a family who loves me and truly missed me while I was away. I came home a much better nurse, because I was challenged to the fullest and rose to the occasion. I came home missing a part of myself that I may never get back because of the things I experienced; however, I know that as an Air Force Officer and a proud OB nurse, I have the skills I need to survive and thrive in any environment.

SUMMARY

Military nurses have been deploying for years, working outside of their traditional clinical roles, and many times out of their comfort zones. Although a significant amount of the preparation military nurses receive to prepare them for battlefield nursing may be formal, much of their training is acquired on the job. Few classroom settings truly prepare nurses for the sights, sounds, and realities of the battlefield. These experiences will continue as long as there are wars, and they will strengthen and define the profession just as previous events have.

REFERENCES

1. Scannell-Desch EA. Lessons learned and advice from Vietnam War nurses: a qualitative study. J Adv Nurs 2005;49(6):600–7.
2. Holder VL. From handmaiden to right hand—World War I—the mud and the blood. AORN J 2004;80(4):652–60, 663–5.
3. Angell D. A war remembered. Aust Nurs J 1998;6(2):28–9.
4. Sarnecky MT. A history of the U.S. Army Nurse Corps. Philadelphia: University of Pennsylvania Press; 1999.
5. Norman EM. We band of angels: the untold story of American nurses trapped on Bataan by the Japanese. New York: Pocket Books; 1999.
6. Griffiths L, Jasper M. Warrior nurse: duality and complementarity of role in the operational environment. J Adv Nurs 2008;61(1):92–9.

Rewards and Challenges of Nursing Wounded Warriors at Landstuhl Regional Medical Center, Germany

Nancy M. Steele, PhD, RNC, WHNP[a],*, Ann Kobiela Ketz, MN[b],
Kathleen D. Martin, MSN, RN, CCRN[c],
Dawn M. Garcia, RN, MHA, CCRN[d],
Shannon Womble, MSN, CCNS, ACNP[e],
Hazel Wright, MSN, MSED, ARNP, RN-BC[f]

KEYWORDS

• Military nurse • Wounded warriors • Trauma • Evacuation

Since March 2003, Landstuhl Regional Medical Center (LRMC) has provided world class, comprehensive, innovative care to more than 45,000 wounded or ill service members from Operations Enduring Freedom (OEF) in Afghanistan and Iraqi Freedom (OIF) in Iraq. They do this while continuing to provide seamless primary care, inpatient care, and treatment to more than 450,000 beneficiaries stationed in Europe,

The opinions or assertions contained herein are solely the views of the authors and should not be construed as official or reflecting the views of the Department of Defense, Department of the Army, and the United States Government.

[a] Nursing Research, Europe Regional Medical Command, Landstuhl Regional Medical Center, CMR 402, Box 726, APO, AE 09180, Landstuhl, Germany

[b] Medical Surgical Unit, Landstuhl Regional Medical Center, CMR 402, Box 512, APO, AE 09180, Landstuhl, Germany

[c] Joint Theater Trauma System, Landstuhl Regional Medical Center, CMR 402, Box 1277, APO, AE 09180, Landstuhl, Germany

[d] Critical Intensive Care Unit, Landstuhl Regional Medical Center, CMR 402, Box 1277, APO, AE 09180, Landstuhl, Germany

[e] Critical Intensive Care Unit, Landstuhl Regional Medical Center, CMR 402, Box 364, APO, AE 09180, Landstuhl, Germany

[f] Staff Development, Education Division, Landstuhl Regional Medical Center, CMR 402, Box 2066, APO, AE 09180, Landstuhl, Germany

* Corresponding author.

E-mail address: nancy.steele@us.army.mil

Nurs Clin N Am 45 (2010) 205–218

doi:10.1016/j.cnur.2010.02.004

0029-6465/10/$ – see front matter. Published by Elsevier Inc.

nursing.theclinics.com

southwest Asia and Africa. A mix of Active Duty and Reserve Army, Air Force, Navy, and civilian nurses work together in this fast-paced environment to stabilize patients and prepare them for return flights to the United States, using specific processes to improve patient outcomes. This article focuses on the unique challenges and rewards of the highly specialized nursing teams who care for the wounded or ill military service members evacuated from OIF and OEF to LRMC. These military service members are referred to as "wounded warriors."

LRMC BACKGROUND

Built in 1953, LRMC is the largest American medical facility located outside the continental United States (CONUS) (**Fig. 1**). Situated in the state of Rheinland-Pfalz in southwest Germany, it is only 3 miles from Ramstein Air Base (RAB). LMRC is strategically located to offer medical care to all military beneficiaries in Europe (Active Duty military, family members, and retirees) and functions as the primary casualty receiving platform for military personnel and civilians injured in Iraq, Afghanistan, and Somalia. In addition to its wartime mission, LRMC is also responsible for primary care and inpatient treatment for approximately 250,000 beneficiaries within Europe and 200,000 US military coalition and civilian contractors from southwest Asia and Africa.[1]

Before 2003, LRMC was considered a low-volume, low-acuity, community-based hospital. This changed abruptly with the onset of the Global War on Terrorism, which resulted in large numbers of medical evacuations from OIF and OEF. Because of LRMC's strategic location in Europe and proximity to RAB, it evolved into a vital element of the military aeromedical evacuation continuum and is now a stopover for transporting the sick and wounded from the battlefields of Iraq and Afghanistan to hospitals in the United States. As a result, LRMC has become a busy, high-volume stabilization center for wounded warriors. On arrival at LRMC, wounded warriors may undergo additional stabilizing surgeries, definitive treatments, and wound care. Once they are able to travel, the US Air Force Aero Medical Evacuation System is used to transport them to the CONUS for further medical, surgical, rehabilitative, and convalescent care by the military and Veteran's Administration (VA) health care systems.[2]

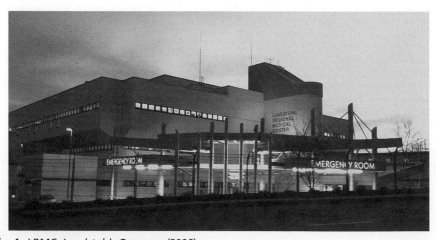

Fig. 1. LRMC, Landstuhl, Germany (2006).

LRMC PATIENT POPULATION

The demographics of the LRMC patient population have changed drastically because of the Global War on Terrorism. According to statistics provided by the Department of Defense, from March 19, 2003, to February 28, 2009, approximately 45,583 individuals were medically evacuated from OIF; 36,106 of these patients had disease or non–battle-related injuries and the remaining 9447 patients had battle-related injuries.[3] The number of patients medically evacuated from OEF for the same period was 9099. The number of disease or non–battle-related injuries and battle-related injuries were 7639 and 1460, respectively.[4]

The numerous medical evacuations from OIF and OEF have resulted in an increase in patient numbers and their level of acuity at LRMC. For example, the average daily intensive care unit (ICU) census has tripled and patient acuity has doubled since 2001.[1] Before OIF and OEF, most ICU patients were older than 50 years and the most common diagnoses were heart disease, lung disease, stroke, and gastrointestinal bleeding. Since the beginning of OIF and OEF, ICU patients have been primarily between 18 and 24 years of age and the most prevalent diagnoses include polytrauma to major body systems, open and closed head injuries, and amputations.[5]

The goal of caring for the wounded warriors is to get them back to the United States for prompt definitive care within 24 to 72 hours. During the Vietnam era, most evacuations from the battlefield to the United States took approximately 45 days.[6] By contrast, from the time of injury of OIF and OEF patients, it takes 24–to 36 hours to transport seriously wounded warriors from the battlefield to LRMC. With today's technology and flight capabilities, most wounded warriors return to a US medical center in less than 5 days.

PREPARING FOR ARRIVAL OF WOUNDED WARRIORS

After OEF and OIF began, nurses' roles changed because LRMC went from being a quiet community hospital to caring for a high volume of acute combat casualty patients evacuated from the war zones.[5] The following scenario depicts a typical day at LRMC as specialized teams of ICU and medical-surgical (med/surg) nurses get ready for the arrival of wounded warriors.

Day-shift nurses have just arrived and are given an update about the 16 patients currently receiving care in the LRMC ICU. The morning report is suddenly interrupted by the ward clerk's loud announcement, "wheels down," which means an incoming flight with wounded warriors and other patients with various illnesses from a combat area has just arrived at RAB and that they will soon be transported to LRMC. Silence fills the room, hearts race, faces lose expression, bodies tense, and all staff members stand ready. Adrenalin levels rise in anticipation of what will transpire in the next few hours. Within seconds, the silence is broken and a multitude of nonverbal and verbal exchanges of information takes place.

The ICU nurses will receive all trauma patients and nontrauma patients requiring mechanical ventilation, invasive monitoring, or vasoactive infusions. They must also prepare a group of 3– to 5 critically injured patients for transport by the Critical Care Air Transport Team (CCATT) to the CONUS. They must make beds available for the incoming wounded warriors. Based on the Patient Movement Records (PMRs), which are available before patients arrive, the nurses must plan to admit 6 new patients from the air transport concurrently with readying patients for transport to the United States. These activities must be accomplished while continuing to care for the 11 critical patients who will remain on the unit.

As mentioned earlier, nursing teams receive clinical information regarding incoming patients through the PMRs. The nurses on each unit receive the PMR the morning of the patient's arrival, usually between 1 and 6 hours before they arrive at LRMC. The PMRs contain vital information about each patient's history, diagnosis, circumstances of injury/illness, treatment course from time of injury to time of evacuation from the combat support hospitals located in the war zones, and potential treatment needs once they arrive at LRMC. The PMR also includes details about medical requirements during the flights, such as equipment required (eg, intravenous pumps, oxygen canisters, chest tube equipment), medications, and whether the patients are ambulatory. The PMRs also provide charge nurses with important information about whether patient should be placed in the ICU or on med/surg units. Because the patients' status may have changed in flight, it can be challenging for charge nurses to compute actual staffing and unit management needs based solely on the PMRs.

The nurses on the med/surg units also receive the announcement for "wheels down," and review them to get a sense of how to proceed to accommodate the new arrivals. Each of the 3 med/surg units can expect to receive up to 5 patients per flight. The nurses strive to anticipate the extent of the patients' injuries to make balanced nursing assignments and obtain the proper equipment, such as wound vacuum-assisted closure (VAC) devices, patient-controlled analgesia (PCA) pumps, and epidural or peripheral nerve-block catheters. Patients are triaged before flight, so that when they arrive at LRMC they are taken directly to a preassigned unit even if their status changed during transport.

After reaching their preassigned unit, all medical evacuation patients are triaged again. Occasionally, they need to be transferred to a different type of unit because of a change in their condition; patients originally destined for the ICU may end up on a med/surg unit or vice versa Because of this possibility, the med/surg charge nurses must be prepared to accept additional patients. On most occasions, charge nurses make every attempt to keep OIF/OEF patients together in the same room. This is based on consistent albeit anecdotal reports of a strong sense of camaraderie between wounded warriors enabling them to provide support to each other.

ARRIVAL OF AIRCRAFT AT RAB

Massive military planes arrive day and night with medical evacuation patients, including wounded warriors, at RAB. The wounded warriors are US soldiers, marines, sailors, airmen, and coalition soldiers who have been fighting on the battlefields in support of OIF and OEF. Air Force cargo planes have been configured and equipped to meet the complex care requirements of patients with different needs, including those who are critically wounded (**Fig. 2**). During the flight, critical patients are cared for by CCATTs, which consist of a critical care nurse, physician, and cardiopulmonary technician. The major responsibilities of the CCATT are to monitor and manage critically ill patients during flight and on American Blue Bird buses called ambuses.[7] Once a plane lands, the CCATTs remain with the patients and assist in transferring them to the ambuses for transport from RAB to LRMC.

There is a large red cross painted on the side of each vehicle to designate that the ambus is being used for military medical unit transport.[8] Like the planes, the ambuses have been constructed to accommodate the litters and special medical equipment requirements of the wounded warriors. To increase the manpower required to transport these patients, the CCATTs are augmented by the Contingency Aeromedical Staging Facility (CASF). CASF teams provide manpower for patient care and movement for all patients transported between the aircraft and LRMC.

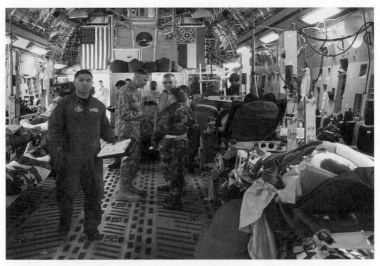

Fig. 2. The inside of an Air Force cargo plane configured and equipped to meet the complex care requirements of en route critical care patients.

The CASF staff are strategically positioned and waiting for the tail of the newly arrived plane to open (**Fig. 3**). The first of 3 ambuses idles, ready to receive the most critically ill and injured patients from the aircraft. The CASF team initiates the transport of the wounded warriors from the aircraft to the medical center. The more critical patients are first carried by litter teams to the ambus, securely strapped to litters affixed to individualized special medical emergency evacuation devices (SMEEDs), which are metal frameworks that act as medical equipment platforms to hold and stabilize individual pieces of equipment, such as ventilators, suction, oxygen cylinders, and multiple intravenous pumps (**Fig. 4**).[9] The team then tends to less critical patients.

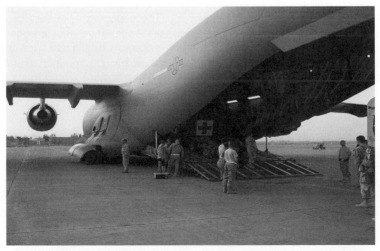

Fig. 3. CASF staff are strategically positioned as the cargo plane's tail opens to allow transport of the wounded warriors out to the awaiting Blue Bird bus.

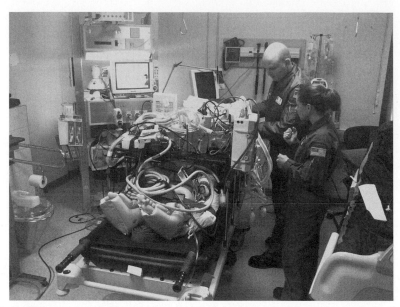

Fig. 4. SMEED acts as a medical equipment platform to hold and stabilize individual pieces of equipment for a transport patient.

There is a flurry of activity as the CCATT members enter the ambus with the first patient. The registered nurse gives a last-minute fentanyl bolus to reduce the patient's pain brought on by the jostling and increased stimulation of yet another transport.[10] The respiratory therapist transfers the patient's oxygen delivery to portable devices. The physician, now on the ambus with the patient, provides increased sedation because the patient's intracranial pressure (ICP) is increased. Meanwhile, the nurse quickly responds to another intubated patient who is waking and trying to sit up; a small bolus of midazolam hydrochloride (Versed) calms him. The last of the CCATT patients are finally secured on the ambus when suddenly another patient monitor alarm is heard. The nurse quickly assesses the situation and increases a patient's dose of norepinephrine bitartrate (Levophed). The sounding of a monitor alarm is not uncommon; nurses must be able to assess the situation and act accordingly. Although the CCATT wants to transport these patients to definitive care as quickly as possible, the ambus must proceed slowly because ground transport is uncomfortable for the patients. After traveling thousands of miles and receiving many hours of continuous lifesaving care, the ambus stops at the emergency department (ED) and the CCATT is met by the LRMC staff.

ARRIVAL OF AMBUSES AT LRMC

Just before the ambuses arrive at the ED, an overhead page sounds at LRMC: "all Department of Nursing manpower report to the emergency department." All available staff from the nursing units are sent to the ED entrance to welcome the wounded warriors and help transport them from the ambus directly to the preassigned patient care units. LRMC critical care nurses, respiratory therapists and other staff, all wearing bright yellow isolation gowns and protective gloves, stand ready.

Minutes slowly go by as the patients are hoisted on their litters by six person teams to a gurney (**Fig. 5**). Some of the patients are still dusty from the sandy environment

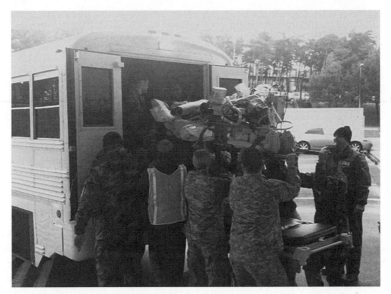

Fig. 5. Outside LRMC's emergency department. A 6-person team hoists a litter carrying a wounded warrior and medical equipment from the bus onto a gurney.

from which they came. The most seriously injured are unloaded first, followed by other litter patients, then those who can ambulate on their own or with crutches. Each warrior is greeted by the chaplain; each arriving warrior is personally acknowledged, whether awake, asleep or in a coma. They are then taken to their awaiting preassigned unit at LRMC.

ARRIVAL OF THE WOUNDED WARRIORS TO PREASSIGNED LRMC UNITS
ICU Placement

A patient report is given to the LRMC nurses by the CCATT members during patient transfer. Six-member teams transfer each patient to their bed. The ICU nurses work together to hook up new equipment and remove the SMEED. A complete assessment is conducted by a nurse, doctor, and respiratory technician. Baseline specimens are obtained and sent to the laboratory. Respiratory technicians prepare to assist with a bronchoscopy on a patient whose oxygen level became dangerously low as he was transferred to the bed. A radiology technician is present to perform portable chest radiographs on all intubated patients. When the patient with the increased ICP arrives, a computerized tomography (CT) technician is called. Nurses quickly multitask; the more experienced nurses provide guidance to novice nurses and those who are new to the unit. In addition to providing direct nursing care, the nurses must ensure that the patients' belongings are with them. The nurses also need to retrieve all records and reports sent from the battlefield medical facility to ensure continuity of treatment.

The ICU patients are in varying stages of sepsis, acute respiratory distress, and multisystem organ failure. These critical patients may need to be supported by advanced modes of ventilation, such as high frequency ventilation or volumetric diffusive respirator (VDR), or lung salvage techniques including inhaled Flolan and nitric oxide, dialysis, surgery, ongoing fluid resuscitation, vasopressors, and multiple antibiotics. Most patients will be ready for transport to a CONUS within 24 to 72 hours after their arrival at LRMC. Others will remain at LRMC until they are stable enough for 10 to 18 hours of air travel. This could require up to 2 weeks of care at LRMC.

Med/Surg Placement

The first several hours of a patient's stay on the med/surg units are hectic. The rooms become crowded as members of multidisciplinary teams (nurses, physicians, respiratory therapists, nutritionists, infection control personnel, and clinical pharmacists) maneuver around each other to triage and provide care. Nursing teams do their best to welcome each patient to the units in the midst of assessments, medical history, and treatments. Often, the long flight on an uncomfortable litter triggers an increased amount of pain and nurses must act quickly to obtain orders for pain medications. Nurses and doctors work closely with anesthesia providers to ensure that a patient's pain is controlled during their stay.[10] Specially trained personnel arrive to screen patients for any signs of traumatic brain injury.[11]

Patients and Families at LRMC

The health care staff focus intently on the patient's health care needs, but most patients are focused on their personal hygiene. After living in an environment of sand storms and extreme temperatures, they want to feel clean; and wash away the sand and blood they carried with them during their long flight from the battlefield. Personal hygiene is secondary, however, to specimen swabs for ruling out multidrug resistant organisms.[12,13] The nurses continually attempt to balance completing their required care tasks and documentation while allowing patients to relax and experience the comforts of their short-term home.

For wounded warriors who remain at LRMC, the government makes arrangements for families to fly to Germany. It is the nursing team's responsibility to initiate this process as soon as the medical team determines the need for a longer stay.

STABILIZATION AND TRANSPORT OUT

Once the patients are settled and the initial paperwork is complete, nurses can focus on other aspects of a patient's care. Because of the speed and efficiency by which wounded warriors are shifted from their point of injury, they may arrive before they have time to realize the emotional effect of their injury or the event that caused it. Staff will facilitate telephone calls home to family and loved ones as soon as possible. The nurses strive to provide patients with the emotional support they need to come to grips with their situation, but often this support is best given by other OEF or OIF patients sharing the room.

Nursing teams also show their support by listening to the warriors' stories and answering questions. They can arrange to meet some of the needs by helping warriors receive some luxury items through various programs. The Chaplain's Closet organizes donations, such as snacks, books, DVDs, phone cards, and some clothing to be distributed among these patients. In addition, personal shoppers from the Army and Air Force Exchange Service, a military department store, get specific requests from patients and are permitted to purchase US$250 worth of clothing and shoes per warrior. Warriors return home with a handmade quilt in honor of their service; these are made through the Quilts of Valor Foundation.[14]

Once a patient is stable, nurses must manage voluminous paperwork to ensure that patients are prepared to fly on the next available flight. Flight lists and itineraries for patients being transferred out are released by the afternoon or evening before the flight. The night-shift nursing team gets everything in order for the patients who will be on the flight, including verifying medications, preparing litters that will be used during the flight, and arranging for equipment that may be needed by the patient. The day-shift nursing team finalizes the flight arrangements, coordinates last-minute changes with the Air Force nurses, and transports patients to buses for transport to the plane that will take them to the CONUS.

Most often, the time between a patient's arrival and departure is short, but the nursing teams work with the warriors to instill a sense of belonging, bolster self-confidence, increase self-reliance, and promote spiritual healing and wellness. Nurses at LRMC feel a sense of gratification in being able to deliver even the smallest gestures that make some warriors smile as they head home on litters, in wheel chairs, on crutches; some badly disfigured, and others bearing invisible wounds and scars.

NURSE STRESSORS

The rewards for the nursing teams are beyond measure, knowing that the care they provide can result in a successful recovery for wounded warriors. Yet, even with these intrinsic rewards, the LRMC nursing teams experience a rollercoaster of emotions as they endeavor to care for the often young, seriously injured patients and listen to the stories of the nonintubated patients and, at times, their families. Similar to other wars, the youth and severity of injury for this patient population adds dramatically to the stressors experienced by the nursing staff caring for them.[5]

The nurses become emotional as they overhear some of the conversations between warriors and families, phrases such as; "I am coming home, just not the same way I left." They join in prayer with chaplains and console families, friends, fellow soldiers, and other nurses, and are present when family and friends first comprehend the severity of a wounded warrior's injuries. Current research demonstrates that LRMC nurses experience significant stress from changes related to the extra work created by deployments and the young age of the returning wounded warriors and the care they require.[5]

DIVERSE MILITARY NURSING STAFF

It is a reward and a challenge for LRMC nurses to work with a diverse group that includes Active Duty and Reserve nurses from the Army, Navy, Air Force and civilian nurses from the Department of Defense. On short notice, each nurse is transported a continent away to live in a foreign country. Despite cultural and educational differences, the nurses form a cohesive team dedicated to caring for the wounded warriors.

There is diversity among the service components and the length of assignments for the nurses at LRMC. Typically, Active Duty Army nurses are assigned for 3 years and Air Force nurses are assigned for 2– to 3 years. Mobilized Reserve nurses, regardless of service, are usually assigned to LRMC for 1 year, but some Reservists on annual training are only at LRMC for 2 to 3 weeks and they may be assigned to positions unrelated to their civilian jobs. This creates a constant turnover in nurses, turnover that is quite different from that experienced in civilian hospitals. For example, in 2007, there was an 80% turnover in LRMC nurses over a 5-day period.[1] This continuous transition can be chaotic, adding numerous challenges and stressors, especially when one group of service nurses departs and the next arrives.

Adding to the challenge from the turnover of nurses, some Active Duty nurses are assigned full time to LRMC, whereas others are assigned to external military units in addition to LRMC. For example, nurses from the 212th Army Combat Support Hospital (CSH) primarily work at LRMC but are also required to spend time training with the 212th CSH, where they travel to field environments and work in portable combat support hospitals that resemble those used in the actual battlefields. This type of training is necessary because the 212th CSH provides care to wounded warriors on the battlefield and nurses assigned to this CSH must be prepared to deploy at any time. The 212th CSH nurses may leave LRMC for days to weeks at a time for field training, leaving LRMC with temporary nurse vacancies and increased workload for the LRMC nurses who remain behind.

Another ongoing nurse staffing challenge is that nurses from the Air Force 435th Medical Support Squadron assigned to LRMC are part of a flight transport team that can be summoned at any given time for emergent medical evacuations. Thus, they may be unavailable and out of the country for days at a time. This constant nurse turnover and turbulence, with loss of experience and specific knowledge of wounded warrior care, remains a perpetual challenge.

Because of the nurse turnover, diversity, and learning requirements, LRMC must continually provide educational programs, competency assessments, and institute standardized processes to ensure safe care to the wounded warriors.

EDUCATION AND COMPETENCIES TO MAINTAIN LEVEL II TRAUMA CENTER STATUS

The increase in number and acuity of combat casualties evacuated from Iraq and Afghanistan necessitated additional assets within LRMC that are typically found in a civilian trauma center. The leadership of LRMC was committed to having LRMC meet the criteria to become a Level II trauma center verified by the American College of Surgeons. The institution was successfully verified in June 2007.[15,16]

This designation has had a significant effect and yielded many positive returns. For example, clinical resources were enhanced and specialized nursing education was enriched by offering courses such as a specific wounded warrior LRMC Trauma Course, the Emergency Nurses' Association Trauma Nurse Care Course (TNCC), Essentials of Critical Care Orientation (ECCO), Advance Trauma Life Support (ATLS), and Advanced Burn Life Support Course (ABLS). The addition of a military version of the Trauma Outcomes and Performance Improvement Course has improved clinical care, as demonstrated by fewer patient complications such as compartment syndrome, infections, and deep vein thrombosis. With fewer complications, there has been a concomitant decline in mortality.[17–19]

As a result of becoming a verified trauma center, LRMC established the first worldwide military Joint Theater Trauma Registry (JTTR),[20–24] a traumatic brain injury screening team,[11] and a robust trauma research program. To maintain the highest level of specialized wounded warrior care, a performance improvement program was established, allowing trauma nurses to collaborate with nurses in other clinical areas to develop policies based on the most current evidence-based practice.[25]

Nurses Training

The advanced technology and changes in the weapons being used in the war, and the complex injuries that result, have pushed the refinement of education and training at LRMC. Training standards have been established to ensure adequate skills preparation and education is provided to the nursing staff with special emphasis on the injury patterns of the wounded warriors at LRMC. In addition, incoming ICU nursing staff members are highly encouraged to have current certifications in Advanced Cardiac Life Support, TNCC, and ABLS.

LRMC nurse educators, managers, and staff nurses are keenly aware of the need to educate nurses at all levels. Adapting training programs to meet the needs of the wounded warrior population lessens stress and allows fuller participation in the management of combat nursing care. The instruction provided in the training programs was altered to enhance staff competency and skill levels necessary to meet the complex care of the wounded warrior. Nursing teams attend didactic sessions, followed by supervised training sessions using technologically advanced simulation mannequins. This training provides nurses with the opportunity to practice trauma nursing skills in a controlled environment.

Because of the high turnover of nursing staff at LRMC, it is a constant challenge to maintain compliance with the American College of Surgeons' standard requirements for a Level II trauma center. To ensure that new nurses are assigned to units that closely match their skill level, the arriving nurses are interviewed individually and placed in units based on their previous experience, education, competency, certification, and licensure. In addition, arriving and departing nurses participate in an orientation process called, Right Seat/Left Seat Hand Off. During this process, the outgoing nurse works along side their nurse replacement for 3 12-hour shifts. Even when there is a major turnover because of the arrival of large groups of Reserve nurses, this education and training process occurs smoothly and efficiently.

Novice nurses are assigned to units where work occurs at a more tempered pace, allowing them time to develop their nursing skills and establish a foundation for acquiring more advanced skills. Competency-based training and performance evaluation are conducted throughout their training, and preceptors assist them in gaining confidence that leads to quality patient care and independent nursing practice.

PERFORMANCE IMPROVEMENT ALONG THE CONTINUUM OF COMBAT CASUALTY CARE

Performance improvement (PI) and evaluation of clinical care are among the cornerstones of the wounded warrior program.[25] Assessment of the care process begins before the patient reaches the doors of LRMC through communication with the clinical care team in the war zone via defense satellite network telephones. Health care providers can view the joint patient tracking application, which has uploaded medical records and encrypted e-mail. Nursing staff monitor trauma activation criteria and compliance with clinical practice guidelines related to the care of the injured patient while they are still en route to LRMC.

An example of this process is the documentation of fluid resuscitation on a flow sheet for burn fluid resuscitation outlined in a military guideline known as the Joint Theater Trauma System (JTTS) Burn Clinical Management Guideline.[17] The burn flow sheet was developed to communicate ongoing fluid resuscitation of burn patients in a more efficient manner.[17–19] As the wounded patient moves along the continuum of care, from the battlefield across 3 continents and 15 times zones, the burn flow sheet is passed from one provider to another, serving as a continuous means of documentation and communication. Clinical performance improved once the burn flow sheet was used routinely; this was reflected by a significant decrease in abdominal compartment syndrome and mortality of burn patients.[23]

PI information such as complications, deficiencies in care, timeliness of care, and adequacy of documentation is communicated to the trauma nurse coordinators on a daily basis. Each weekday morning, care provided for all multisystem trauma patients is reviewed. Individuals involved in the review include the trauma program director, trauma nurse director, trauma PI nurse, the postcall physician from the ICU, and trauma nurse coordinators. This review is an opportunity to capture complications and adverse events as soon as they occur, keep the key trauma leadership apprised of potential system issues, and ensure optimal care for these complex wounded warriors. Examples of issues that may be communicated to the trauma nurse coordinators include missed injuries, delays in diagnosis, preventable complications, equipment failures, and delays in obtaining documentation or radiographs from the various forward operating bases and CSHs in the war zone.

On the multinational level, the LRMC trauma team initiated, and is also actively involved in a unique PI process through a weekly video teleconference (VTC).[26] The VTC includes video or audio participation of the clinical team along the continuum of care of the evacuation chain. This lengthy clinical chain includes the field hospitals and CSHs located in the battlefield zones, LRMC, and the 4 stateside treatment facilities that receive patients from OIF/OEF (Walter Reed Army Medical Center, National Naval Medical Center Bethesda, Brooke Army Medical Center, and Wilford Hall Medical Center) and the Tampa Veterans Administration Polyclinic Rehabilitation Facility.

During the video teleconference, open discussions occur about communication, clinical care, complications, transport and equipment, as well as opportunities to enhance care. Intensive care nurses, trauma nurse coordinators, other specialty unit nurses, and all members of the LRMC trauma team participate in the VTC. Trauma nurse coordinators from other facilities along the entire evacuation chain communicate in real time with the LRMC trauma nurse coordinators to share practice guidelines, enhancements in care, and lessons learned.[26] There is also a monthly JTTS nursing teleconference that centers on issues regarding combat casualty patients across the continuum, with a focus on optimizing nursing care.

PI opportunities are entered into the JTTR by the trauma nurse coordinators on a daily basis. The JTTR is a complex database that has more than 400 data elements and a database to track and trend PI issues.[20,21,23] For instance, the JTTR enables staff to assess complications and variances from standards of care and compliance even as the warriors are en route via air medical evacuation, during their stay at LRMC, and during transit to the CONUS. The trauma nurse coordinators validate all identified complications and events by communicating with the bedside nurses and other providers. The primary review of performance issues may immediately change a patient's plan of care. One example is an oversight in ordering deep vein thrombosis prophylaxis for a patient on admission to the ward/unit. Secondary review allows validation of identified issues and triggers. Additional information is collected, analyzed, validated, and in some cases, closure of the issue may be reached. Many concerns may be forwarded to the ICU nurse managers for follow up and corrective action. System issues are reviewed in the Trauma Operational Process Performance Committee.[22]

ONGOING COLLABORATION OF NURSE TEAMS

The military trauma transport system, although analogous to the civilian trauma system model is challenged because of the rapid movement of patients among military treatment facilities and providers across 3 continents and several time zones, and there is an increased likelihood for miscommunication in this large system. Ongoing collaboration and networking among trauma nurse coordinators and unit-specific nurses within the JTTS facilitate much needed consistency in care across the combat casualty continuum.

SUMMARY

LRMC is a vital stop along the road to recovery for wounded warriors. The organized process involves a complex compilation of medical records, transports, numerous providers, and multiple handoffs. Nursing teams at LRMC feel compelled to do their best for the men and women who are sacrificing their lives for our freedom; taking care of the wounded warrior population can be extremely rewarding for the LRMC nursing teams. These nurses provide exceptional care in challenging conditions while maintaining the standards of care found in the best civilian trauma centers. The nurses of LRMC have set the standard of nursing care for the modern battlefield and will continue to foster advances in military trauma nursing.

REFERENCES

1. Fang R, Pruitt VM, Dorlac GR, et al. Critical care at Landstuhl Regional Medical Center. Crit Care Med 2008;36(7):S383–7.
2. Moore EE, Knudsen MM, Schwab CW, et al. Military-civilian collaboration in trauma care and the senior visiting surgeon program. N Engl J Med 2007; 357(26):2723–7.
3. Defense Manpower Data Center. Department of Defense Web site. Available at: http://siadapp.dmdc.osd.mil/personnel/CASUALTY/OIF-Total.pdf. Accessed July 14, 2009.
4. Coalition casualty count. Available at: http://www.icasualties.org. Accessed July 11, 2009.
5. Kenny DJ, Hull MS. Critical care nurses' experiences caring for the casualties of war evacuated from the front line: lessons learned and needs identified. Crit Care Nurs Clin North Am 2008;20(1):41–9.
6. Tenuta JJ. From the battlefields to the States: the road to recovery. The role of Landstuhl Regional Medical Center in U.S. military casualty care. J Am Acad Orthop Surg 2006;14(10):S45–7.
7. Collins ST. Emergency medical support units to critical care transport teams in Iraq. Crit Care Nurs Clin North Am 2008;20:1–11.
8. Geneva Convention. Red Cross and Red Crescent Flags Web sites. Available at: http://flagspot.net/flags/int-red.html. Accessed July 12, 2009.
9. Special Medical Emergency Evacuation Device (SMEED). Department of Defense U.S. Army Institute of Surgical Research publication. Available at: http://www.flcmidatlantic.org/pdf/publications/Special_Medical_Emergency_evacuationdevice.pdf. Accessed April 12, 2009.
10. Military Advanced Regional Anesthesia and Analgesia Handbook. Chapter 20: Air transport of the critically injured patient: controlling pain during transport and flight. Army Regional Anesthesia & Pain Management Initiative Web site. Available at: http://www.arapmi.org/maraa-book-project.html. Accessed May 5, 2009.
11. Dempsey KE, Dorlac WC, Martin K, et al. Landstuhl Regional Medical Center: traumatic brain injury screening program. J Trauma Nurs 2009;16(1):6–7, 10–12.
12. Griffith ME, Lazarus DR, Mann PB, et al. Acinetobacter skin carriage among US Army soldiers deployed in Iraq. Infect Control Hosp Epidemiol 2007;28(6):720–2.
13. Cilento B, Culbertson CL, Gallagher AL. Multidisciplinary approach to infection control for combat casualties. J Trauma Nurs 2008;15(4):197–9.
14. The Quilts of Valor Foundation. Available at: http://www.qovf.org/. Accessed May 15, 2009.
15. American College of Surgeons: Trauma Centers. Verified trauma centers. Available at: http://www.facs.org/trauma/verified.html. Accessed April 10, 2009.
16. Martin K, Dorlac W, Flaherty S, et al. Development of military model trauma center and level II trauma center verification at an echelon 4 military treatment facility.

Poster presentation at 11th Annual Conference Society of Trauma Nurses. New Orleans (LA), April 9, 2008.

17. Joint Theater Trauma System clinical practice guideline: burns. United States Army Institute of Surgical Research Medical Research and Materiel Command Web site. Available at: http://www.usaisr.amedd.army.mil/cpgs/Burn0811.pdf. Accessed April 14, 2009.

18. Chung LL, Blackbourne LH, Wolf SE, et al. Evolution of burn resuscitation in operation Iraqi Freedom. J Burn Care Res 2006;27(5):606–11.

19. Renz EM, Cancio LC, Barillo DJ, et al. Long-range transport of war-related burn casualties. J Trauma 2008;64(2):S136–45.

20. Fecura SE Jr, Martin CM, Martin KD, et al. Nurses role in the Joint Theater Trauma System. J Trauma Nurs 2008;15(4):170–3.

21. Glenn MA, Martin KD, Monzon D, et al. Implementation of a combat casualty trauma registry. J Trauma Nurs 2008;15(4):181–4.

22. Martin K, Flaherty S, Fang R, et al. Concurrent PI and the Joint Theater Trauma System: tools that improve the combat casualty care system. Poster presentation at American Association for the Surgery of Trauma Annual Conference. Maui (HI), September 23, 2008.

23. Holcomb JB, McMullin NR, Pearse L, et al. Causes of death in U.S. Special Operations Forces in the global war on terrorism: 2001–2004. Ann Surg 2007;245(6): 986–91.

24. Spott M, Holcomb J, Jenkins D, et al. Development of an international trauma registry - the military experience. Poster presentation at 11th Annual Conference Society of Trauma Nurses. New Orleans (LA), April 9, 2008.

25. De Jong MJ, Martin JD, Huddleson M, et al. Performance improvement on the battlefield. J Trauma Nurs 2008;15(4):174–80.

26. American College of Surgeons Committee on Trauma. Resources for optimal care of the injured patient. Chicago: American College of Surgeons; 2006.

Implementing Basic Infection Control Practices in Disaster Situations

Elizabeth A.P. Vane, MSN, RN[a],*, Thomas G. Winthrop, MSN, RN[b],
Leonardo M. Martinez, MPH, RN[c]

KEYWORDS

- Basic infection control and prevention • Disaster planning
- Disease transmission • Surveillance program • Military

Infections, troublesome in even optimal health care environments, can be a source of serious and persistent concern for the local population and health care workers during a disaster. Because disaster situations often involve power outages, shortages of water and food, and damage to critical infrastructure, cutting off access to communications and travel (eg, destruction of roads and interruption of communications networks), it is critical to have basic infection control practices in place in order to contain the spread of disease and improve conditions more immediately for those affected. Toole and Waldman[1] define a disaster as "a relatively acute situation created by manmade, geophysical, weather-related, or biological events that adversely impacts on the health and economic well-being of a community to an extent that exceeds the local coping capacity." Basic infection control, as opposed to a more comprehensive program, is essential in disaster management because the procedures can be implemented by both the provider and the recipient. Historically, the United States military has gained extensive knowledge about infection control through its experience managing diseases in different geographical areas and climates, while dealing with cultural and political scenarios that directly affect the delivery of health care.

The opinions or assertions contained herein are solely the views of the authors and should not be construed as official or reflecting the views of the Department of Defense or United States Government.
[a] Perioperative Clinical Nurse Specialist Program, Graduate School of Nursing, Uniformed Services University of the Health Sciences, Graduate School of Nursing, Building E, 4301 Jones Bridge Road, Bethesda, MD 20814, USA
[b] Perioperative Services, Walter Reed Army Medical Center, Washington, DC 20307, USA
[c] Preventive Medicine, DeWitt Health Care Network, Fort Belvoir, VA 22060-5901, USA
* Corresponding author.
E-mail address: Elizabeth.vane@usuhs.mil

HISTORICAL PERSPECTIVES ON INFECTION CONTROL
A Second Century Approach to Disease Management

The Bible refers to a range of disasters from floods and locusts to epidemics. Persian, Egyptian, Greek, and Roman physicians focused principally on medicinal efforts for wound management. Many of the therapies involved cleansing wounds with everything from water, beer, donkey feces, and grease to various herbal concoctions.[2] Galen of Pergamum wrote a large body of work on wound management related to Roman gladiators but erroneously identified pus as a positive factor, an assertion that impeded infection control practices for centuries.[2]

The Black Death of the Fourteenth Century

The Black Death plague that occurred in medieval Europe from 1347 to 1351 is an excellent example of both mismanagement and proper management of infection. Initially, populations were powerless against the onslaught of the epidemic. The Black Death, now thought to be an outbreak of the bubonic plague, killed one third of Europe's population.[3] Eventually, basic principles of isolation, improved sanitation, and vector control were used to limit the spread of the disease.

Disease Management in Nineteenth Century Military Operations

Over centuries, a systematic approach to infection control gradually developed based on knowledge gained from military operations. Military campaigns brought with them the need for wound and disease management.

As chief nurse for the military hospital in Scutari, Turkey, during the Crimean War (1854 to 1856), Florence Nightingale learned that "improved sanitary conditions in military hospitals and barracks could sharply cut the death rate and save thousands of lives".[4] Six months after arriving at a British hospital in Scutari, her efforts to improve the laundry, kitchen, and hygiene of staff and patients, and the way supplies were gathered contributed to reducing the mortality rate of wounded soldiers dying from disease from 42.7% to 2.2%.[4]

During the American Civil War (1861 to 1865), practices in disease management were further advanced, including the use of general anesthetics for surgery, delay of amputation to reduce shock, bromine to prevent gangrene, carbolic acid and sodium hypochlorite to treat gangrene, avoidance of surgery for penetrating abdominal wounds, and maggot therapy.[2]

During the Spanish-American War of 1898, yellow fever caused the deaths of thousands of soldiers resulting in the US Army sending a team to Cuba to investigate the epidemic. At that time, it was believed that yellow fever was spread on clothing of infected patients and from person-to-person contact. However, in 1900, a US Army physician, Major Walter Reed, discovered that mosquitoes were the carriers of the deadly fever.[5] Using epidemiological principles for controlling mosquitoes, Major Reed ensured that their breeding grounds were drained and screens were placed on houses.

Soon after, interest peaked in controlling malaria as well as yellow fever so the US Army could build the Panama Canal to join the Caribbean Sea to the Pacific Ocean. In 1904, the Sanitary Department was formed with US Army Colonel William Crawford Gorgas as the first chief sanitary officer. Colonel Gorgas was an expert in construction sanitation, an important skill because mosquitoes also carried malaria.[6] Dr Gorgas developed a program to (1) drain areas where mosquitoes were breeding, (2) add larvicide oil to kill mosquito larvae in swamps that could not be drained, (3) cut brush and grass near homes to 1 foot high, (4) distribute the medication quinine to workers, and

(5) build screens onto all government buildings.[6] Building the Panama Canal was a huge and difficult construction project. In addition, the project demonstrated how well diseases such as yellow fever and malaria could be controlled.

The Twentieth Century Faces an Evolving Disease Threat

In 1915, poison gas was used during attacks in World War I,[7] adding a new dimension to disaster and disease management. Improved sanitation and vector control could not contain the harm inflicted by poisonous gas.

As World War I was ending, the first flu pandemic occurred from 1918 to 1919, killing 40 million people around the world.[8] On December 28, 1918, the *Journal of the American Medical Association* printed the following:

> *The 1918 has gone: a year momentous as the termination of the most cruel war in the annals of the human race: a year which marked, the end at least for a time, of man's destruction of man; unfortunately a year in which developed a most fatal infectious disease causing the death of hundreds of thousands of human beings. Medical science for four and one-half years devoted itself to putting men on the firing line and keeping them there. Now it must turn with its whole might to combating the greatest enemy of all—infectious disease.*[8]

Events from World War I and the 1918 influenza pandemic prompted scientists to develop new applications for germ theory, antiseptic surgical techniques, vaccines and sanitary measures to prevent and treat infectious diseases. Public health departments were also better able to distribute information about the spread of diseases and how to break the deadly chain of infection transmission.

It was not until 1980 that the Association for Practitioners in Infection Control, which later became the Association for Professionals in Infection Control and Epidemiology, developed standards in the following specific areas for infection control practice: epidemiology; microbiology; infectious diseases; sterilization, disinfection, and sanitation; patient care; education; management and communication; and employee health.[9] This multifaceted approach is critically important to the success of infection control efforts during disasters. It offers providers a framework for attending to basic infection control measures, detecting problem areas early, and implementing countermeasures to control the spread of disease.

Infection control and the threat of terror in the twenty-first century

Today, infection control measures must take into account the threat of terrorism and the potential for a range of terror attacks—chemical, biological, and nuclear—and a range of materials from explosives to radiation. Biological attacks are particularly insidious as they may be hard to detect. Prompt reporting and surveillance practices are critical to detecting and containing a biological attack.

Recently, a biological scenario was used for a mass casualty simulation in a large US city. During the simulation, patients presented to various military and civilian hospitals in the area with nonspecific symptoms. The scenario played out over 4 days until a pattern was discovered, after which a biological alert was issued. The potential exposures from the time of the initial presentations until diagnosis and alert are indicative of the danger associated with a bioterrorism event. Clinically, the mitigating factor in diminishing the severity of such an attack depends on how well responders such as health care workers and hospital staff practice basic infection control policies. Biological warfare using an agent such as smallpox would "dwarf any previous infection control concern."[10]

PRACTICAL ISSUES IN DISASTER MANAGEMENT

Nothing is easy during disasters—from accessing the area and dealing with logistics to coming to the aid of a population in need of, or lacking in, basic amenities and services. For example, interruptions to power would not only create issues with visibility and food refrigeration but would disrupt communication because telephones, computers, radios, and televisions would be affected as well. There could also be issues with passable roads, running water, and safe places to live and work. Add to that possible threats to safety, and the challenges of effectively addressing infection control issues are monumental.

MANAGING DISASTERS IN TIMES OF FAMINE AND DISEASE

During the past 20 years, military planners have had much experience with disaster management. This experience has been rich in lessons learned, from both things that were done well and things that could have been done better. For instance, an incident in Somalia in the early 1990s illustrates the myriad of problems caregivers face in disaster management. The capital, Mogadishu, is a city of more than two million people, many of whom live without electricity or running water. Warring groups had destroyed the local agriculture, which led to mass starvation. When other countries responded by sending food to Somalia, local leaders intercepted the food to barter for weapons. This led to millions of displaced refugees, hundreds of thousands of casualties, as well as endemic disease resulting from malnutrition and lack of proper sanitation. In 1992, the United Nations began an operation to help the Somali people receive food; however, what began as a mission to bring food to starving Somali ended in military battle. During the fighting, military health care providers were routinely exposed to a multitude of contagious diseases including tuberculosis, chicken pox, and other illnesses that are contained in Western society.

Climate, Water, and Other Disease Management Considerations

Climate is another main consideration in controlling infections during disasters. Whereas temperatures range from 70°F to 90°F in Mogadishu,[11] the Balkan countries experience a hot summer and a cold winter climate. For example, due to snow, mud, and cold weather, the military hospital established in Tuzla, Bosnia, in support of the Implementation Force from 1995 to 1996, had to be built on wooden platforms. This created challenges for maintaining basic cleanliness of the facility.

Another classic infection control issue involves disposing of human waste. To the left of the makeshift latrine shown in the center of **Fig. 1** is a "burn pot"—a metal drum cut in half. When the metal drum was full, the contents had to be burned. To the right of the latrine is the hand-washing station—a bar of soap is hanging in a nylon stocking on the side of a 5-gallon container filled with water. During winter, temperatures were cold enough to freeze the water at the hand-washing station, making basic hygiene difficult.

Disaster relief usually involves a coalition of military, civilian, and United Nations groups. Even when these relief workers are able to occupy fixed facilities, problems may arise. For example, buildings such as warehouses are often used as makeshift hospitals. These buildings typically have major water and sewage problems, along with indigent arthropod, rodent, and bird infestations. Supplying water and electricity to fixed facilities is also problematic. The task is often more difficult for US-based relief groups, which, for instance, may have 110-volt power equipment instead of the 220-volt power equipment commonly used overseas.

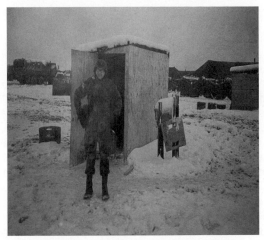

Fig. 1. Makeshift latrine with "burn pot" on left. Hand-washing station consists of a bar of soap in a nylon hose, hanging on the side of a frozen 5-gallon water container (Bosnia, 1996).

An equally critical consideration in any relief contingency is the people, their culture, their health care beliefs, and how they live. A prior knowledge of the people who are affected can inform the planning of effective approaches for infection control.

THE ROLE OF SUBCONTRACTORS AND FOREIGN HEALTH RESPONDERS IN DISEASE CONTROL

In many parts of the world, infection control does not receive the attention it does in more developed countries. However, this thinking is not necessarily shared by care providers from countries where antibiotics are commonly used and water is treated. Foreign responders, by contrast, may have a large contingent of subcontractors who come from countries that do not have readily accessible treated water and antibiotics. These subcontractors add another component to infection control in that they may be poorly screened for health issues themselves, which may pose a significant risk to other health providers as well as the local population. Toole and Waldman[1] found that "front line relief workers in complex emergencies are often volunteers recruited by Non-Government Relief Organizations who sometimes lack specific training and experience in emergency relief." These workers may be working in food service, acting as interpreters for patients, or providing basic housekeeping activities. Failure to adequately screen these individuals may lead to unexpected outbreaks.

FEAR OF A GLOBAL DISEASE OUTBREAK

A new threat, H1N1, or swine flu, emerged quickly and unexpectedly in 2009. It was a new virus for which there were low levels of immunity in the younger population.[12] In addition, the risk of transporting a virus, drug-resistant organism or an exotic disease from one country to another or from one disaster site to another is a serious matter. Moreover, the mobility of today's populations can make the worldwide spread of an undetected disease possible very quickly.[13] Reducing the threat of transporting a virus may be done by screening people on entry or exit of a destination or by initiating modified forms of decontamination.

On a global level, there is the potential for highly pathogenic avian influenza (HPAI) to exert a worldwide effect. The main strategy to combat HPAI is aimed at minimizing the threat at the source.[14] However, the potential for an HPAI outbreak due to the mobility and migration patterns of birds presents health planners with a potentially lethal scenario. Planning for military deployments includes setting contingencies for such epidemics. This is especially true in settings such as Iraq and Afghanistan where the environment can include sandstorms, extreme heat and cold, working in tents, and questionable sanitation facilities. Responding to such an event would primarily center on providing a large facility or tent to house patients suspected of having avian flu. Unused buildings or tents with water and sanitation equipment could be quickly converted into isolation and treatment centers. Surveillance and reporting are critical factors in containing an outbreak, but this often is not possible in some countries.

The importance of infection control and prevention grows in both scale and scope when practiced outside the hospital setting. So-called basic principles are quite challenging to implement. Broader training in infection control practices is recommended for personnel responding to disaster situations.[15] However, because disasters are unpredictable events, it is likely that personnel who would be involved in responding to the next disaster would lack this broader training. Even with the broad disaster response experience among military personnel, infection control knowledge is likely to vary among responders.

A MACRO- VERSUS MICROLEVEL APPROACH TO INFECTION CONTROL

Response to disasters may be analyzed by a two-fold approach—a macro or strategic approach, which is broad, and a more detailed micro or operational approach. It is important to understand the relationship between the macro- and microlevels of disaster planning. At the macrolevel, a strategic approach centers on the disaster management of infection control to include a complete analysis of all environmental conditions, the risk factors for that event and region—such as vector prevalence, and available resources. The micro or operational level is focused on executing what should be a well-prepared disaster response plan.

The macrolevel concerns the overall response and implementation of a disaster plan. This is ongoing and conducted by professionals using all resources available. In the United States, the macrolevel assessment of disasters occurs at the federal level. The significance and coordination of efforts are accomplished through the National Response Plan.[16] The highest level event is categorized as an Incident of National Significance; it falls under the purview of the National Response Plan. Such a response is coordinated under the National Incident Management System, which implements "federal, state, local, tribal, private sector, and non-governmental entities to save lives, minimize damage, and provide the basis for long-term community recovery and mitigation of activities."[16] Although avian flu and H1N1 are a real threat today, the rise of terrorism around the globe and the threat of a nuclear, chemical, biological, radiological, or high-yield explosive incident magnifies the importance of macrolevel planning.

At the microlevel, disaster response is coordinated by the state or local government depending on the severity of the event. The magnitude of the response is determined by parameters set by Homeland Security Presidential Directive/HSPS-5.[16] The operational plan at the microlevel is formulated by bringing together all available assets in the area of operations. Preventive medicine, infection control, infectious disease, veterinary and medical, and nursing personnel all play a part in developing a coherent plan to limit the spread of disease and protect the population. In many instances, coordination among available resources simply does not occur. For instance, many nongovernment relief organizations do not always coordinate their activities or experience with the larger operation. However, when these groups participate in the planning, they lend an invaluable source of expertise. This was the case in humanitarian efforts in Somalia and Bosnia, for example. It also is reportedly current practice in the Middle East.

Recent examples of microlevel planning include efforts to control disease at Tallil Air Base, Iraq. Characteristic of disaster events or deployments is the continuous influx and departure of personnel. The mobility of personnel increases the potential for missing critical signs of an impending infection control problem. The preventive medicine (PM) officer on the air base assessed the situation and realized that the task of protecting the personnel demanded a more focused approach. The first action was to determine who could assist. Assistance was found from personnel in other units and from coalition forces. For example, the PM officer implemented a program to protect the military personnel assigned to the area by bringing together the infection prevention and control nurse, a PM technician from another US military unit, the Veterinarian Detachments, an Australian infectious disease physician, and a Romanian NBC (nuclear, biological, chemical) decontamination unit. These actions were highly effective. An outbreak of meningitis in the Iraqi Army camp was contained, a sexually transmitted disease problem was identified and eliminated, and a hospital interpreter was screened and treated for tuberculosis. In addition, the veterinarians dealt with an increasing intrusion of wild animals onto the base that could have posed a serious health issue for the base population.

SUCCESSFUL INFECTION MANAGEMENT

In the deployed military setting, there are three focal points for infection control and prevention: sanitary practices, disinfection and sterilization, and isolation.[10] According to Roup and Kelley,[10] "successful infection control programs usually have an active multidisciplinary infection control committee; proactive surveillance; effective methods for isolating patients and specimens that pose a risk to others; an occupational health program; policies regarding antibiotic use, aseptic technique, and facility sanitation; and access to at least basic microbiological laboratory support." It is at this point in the disaster response that theory and planning transitions to practical application of basic infection control techniques. The success of an operation cannot be achieved simply by the implementation of an infection control program. A successful infection control program can only be accomplished by strict monitoring of the program basics. The use of a checklist, which focuses unit or operational level providers on the basics, is the key to successfully limiting the spread of infectious diseases in a disaster situation.

CHECKLISTS AND FOUR PRINCIPLES OF INFECTION CONTROL
Checklists in Disaster Response Planning

Fig. 2 is a checklist that was developed by the US Army nurses of the 212th Mobile Army Surgical Hospital (MASH) in Bosnia in 1996 and has been improved upon through multiple deployments to the present. This checklist incorporates the four principles of infection control: (1) education, (2) monitoring, (3) surveillance, and (4) reporting, and provides for a mechanism to focus on the essentials.

REVIEWER: _____   DATE:_____

	Day	Evening	Night
Education			
In-service trainings			
Journal articles			
Surveillance			
Employee health screen (including exposures)			
Inoculations			
TB screen			
Monitoring			
Engineering			
Sharps container (available/full)			
Hand-washing station (soap available)			
Eye wash station			
Floor free of litter			
Linen bags turned in (clean/dirty are separated)			
Sterile/unsterile supplies separated			
Eating area clean			
Regulated medical waste disposed of correctly			
Trash bags with liners			
Areas clean			
Spill kits available			
Clinical			
Sterilization records complete (biological log)			
Decontamination testing			
Challenge packs in loads			
Universal precautions			
PPE compliance			
Hand washing			
Reporting			
All breaks in sterility			
Reportable diseases			
Needle/sharps injuries			

Fig. 2. Infection Control Monitoring Tool for Deployed Settings.

Checklists, which focus on basic yet essential acts, have been effective in many areas for ensuring adherence to safety guidelines and are becoming an integral part of the health care environment. Hayes and colleagues[17] recently completed a study using checklists to minimize errors in surgery and found that "a checklist-based program was associated with a significant decline in the rate of complications and death from surgery in a diverse group of institutions around the world ... Applied on a global basis, this checklist program has a potential to prevent large numbers of deaths and disabling complications."[17]

Checklists differ from infection control inspection lists, which are common in health care. Both types of lists allow providers to monitor and report data crucial to infection control practices. However, although thorough, an inspection list is not easily implemented in a disaster situation. Nor does it cover the contingencies associated with groups of responders with varying degrees of infection control knowledge.

A checklist could easily be adapted to include specific areas that comprise the response team's responsibility. For example, a more detailed checklist could be adapted for surgical instrument processing and sterilization to guide stocking reusable supplies in a disaster scenario. Effort should be made to conform care processes in disaster conditions as closely as possible to those normally found in hospitals. This again involves careful preplanning. Great strides have been made in technology to replicate processes for unconventional hospital environments including everything from portable sterilizers to easily performed quality assurance tests. In addition, the introduction of new advances, especially in testing methods, such as the ability to test water quality and decontamination effectiveness, enables a unit-level manager to tailor infection control processes to the most basic operational level. The basic disaster infection control checklist is disseminated to all areas within the hospital so each area can add critical parameters to the list to make a more effective program.

Although it is easy to add parameters to a checklist to address specific issues, it is important to keep to the basics. The effectiveness of an infection control program is correlated with the number of parameters monitored. In disaster situations, health care workers are already operating under a high level of stress. Adhering to the basics helps workers focus on the priorities of the infection control program while still allowing them to perform their primary jobs. Having reliable reference material to refer to, teach from, and consult will help all staff to focus on the priority tasks.

Communication is the foundation for basic infection control. It is a mechanism to initiate action, whether it be reporting a finding or warning of a potential problem or shortfall. Breaks in communication equate to failure to take action. They lead to the possibility of a negative outcome such as propagating infections by misusing cleaning products, diluting chemical disinfectants incorrectly, failing to recognize symptoms of a contagious disease process, and deviating from standard infection control procedures.

Finally, what are the consequences of failing to implement and enforce adherence to basic infection control practices? Staff may merely fill out the checklist without due diligence. The point is not to fill out a checklist but to use it to remind and reinforce proper infection control and also to use as an evaluation tool to assess and reassess proper procedures. The bioterrorism example cited earlier illustrates the importance of having sound infection control procedures that are in place and that are observed.

Educating Infection Control Personnel

Education is vital to the effectiveness of deployed providers and the infection control program they help to carry out. Roup and Kelley[10] concluded that "the underpinning of a successful [infection control] program is regular education and communication. Infection control must be given emphasis and responsible personnel to be successful." **Fig. 2** lists two educational opportunities: staff in-services and the sharing of journal articles. Education can be focused on tailoring these activities to the specific situation. Emphasis should include a range of topics from basic hand washing to ensuring the providers have an understanding of the diseases prevalent in the area. Educational materials can be developed and distributed to all groups providing support.

An example from a military operation best illustrates a successful outcome in this area. The Public Health officer for the 28th Combat Support Hospital in Mosul, Iraq, routinely visited contractor facilities to educate and relay important infection control practices. Presentations about *Acinetobacter* were provided to reinforce information that many may have missed in briefings prior to deployment to Iraq. *Acinetobacter* is a bacterium commonly found in soil and water and has been problematic in the wounds of service members returning from the war zone.

For a disaster scenario, where the situation is not normal, education may also involve emphasizing to staff the importance of "doing the best you can for the most people" because disaster situations may not allow responders to handle individual patients. Rather, following the practices that are best for the population as a whole can be the most effective way of containing infection. Identifying individuals who are responsible for the infection control program in their unique clinical area can be very helpful in making the program a success.

The Use of Monitoring in Infection Control

Monitoring, a key component of infection control, can be best understand through its engineering and clinical components (see **Fig. 2**) to make the process more manageable and intuitive. It may be easier to solve an engineering problem than a clinical one; personal health care practices are harder to change if not monitored closely. Critical practices of hand washing and disposal of hazardous waste, for example, may be neglected. In the chaos of a disaster, simple, routine practices can be forgotten. The checklist assists in monitoring by serving as reminders to health care workers of containment behaviors such as hand washing and the necessity of items such as trash bags, spill kits, eyewash stations, and water. For instance, the United Nations High Commissioner for Refugees recommends providing a minimum of 20 liters of potable water per person per day for domestic needs—cooking, drinking, and bathing.[18] Not every disaster situation will involve refugees, but the concept of how much water is needed for basic needs can be elusive. Water needs are an essential consideration for personal hygiene and hand-washing practices. Additionally, water needed for cleaning and sterilizing surgical instruments and other equipment and the demand for water is increased.

Employing Surveillance in Disaster Control

Not only must infection control practices be observed for patients in disaster scenarios, but healthcare providers must also know how to protect themselves. It is common for health care providers to ignore basic policies such as choosing not to eat at a co-located nongovernment relief organizations facility or declining food and drink given by a local worker. There is rarely a military operation where someone is not diagnosed with salmonella or another exotic disease acquired from disregarding standard policy. A good example of surveying at the worker level can also be found in Mosul. In 2007, a third-party subcontractor was admitted to the emergency room and eventually diagnosed with chicken pox. The workers he was housed with were quickly quarantined. Upon further investigation, it was discovered that a large group of these contractors were recently imported from another country in which chicken pox was prevalent during that season. This led to a review of the hiring practices along with health screening of workers prior to deployment from Kuwait.

Reporting Infections in a Disaster

Reporting is the last of the four major infection control basics. It includes accounting for everything from needle sticks and breaks in aseptic practice to exposure to tuberculosis. Any potential for disease spread must be identified early and addressed appropriately. Trained infection control professionals cannot be effective if they do not have necessary information. Seemingly insignificant matters may have far-reaching consequences.

Another aspect of reporting involves the Health Insurance Portability and Accountability Act (HIPAA). Many hospitals in the United States do not have the communications infrastructure to share necessary information between facilities with regard to medical records, patient privacy, and security issues, even in trauma situations.[19] The situation can be even more complex when dealing with disasters outside the

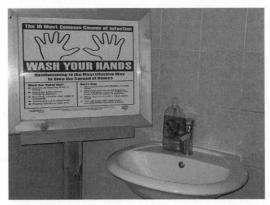

Fig. 3. Hand-washing instructions in military dining facility (Iraq, 2007) The instructions, which are in use today, are intended to transcend cultural and language barriers.

United States. The ability to communicate patient information between hospitals and providers is crucial when dealing with matters of infection prevention and control.

CURRENT ADVANCES IN INFECTION CONTROL PRACTICES

Advances have been made in infection control practices and largely involve establishment of standards of care. These standards have been adopted by the US military. Rather than the latrine, burn pot, and improvised hand-washing station shown in **Fig. 1**, the military now deploys with commercial portable toilets equipped with waterless hand scrub dispensers attached to the wall. Procedures are also in place to routinely check hand scrub dispensers to make sure they are filled. This is a simple but important aspect of infection control. Another current infection control measure now part of standard practice in the military environments is the placement of multiple hand-washing stations at entrances to military dining facilities. A full-time attendant not only checks for supplies and cleanliness but also, and more importantly, ensures that everyone who enters washes their hands before joining the food line. **Fig. 3** displays a sign for hand washing that transcends culture and language. The cardinal tenet of infection control practice is hand washing, and this practice must be brought down to the most rudimentary level for all to understand.

SUMMARY

Once a disaster has occurred, the possibility of an epidemic is prevalent. An emergency relief program that can be immediately put into practice is imperative and would involve (1) establishing surveillance processes; (2) developing standard case management protocol agreement on policies for prevention—including vaccination and prophylaxis—along with environmental management plans; (3) having reserve supplies of essential medical materials, including intravenous solutions and antibodies, and sources of relevant vaccines; (4) identifying treatment sites, triage systems, training needs, and expert assistance for epidemic investigation along with a laboratory to confirm index cases of epidemic disease; and (5) quick implementation of community education and evaluation programs.[1] Implementing infection control practices involves a two-fold approach—a macro or strategic approach and a micro or operational approach. At the strategic level, overall planning and resource management determine the effectiveness of the response. This includes compiling environmental analyses and stockpiling supplies including hand-washing supplies and equipment for laboratory testing. The success of rapidly mobilizing and deploying assorted relief groups depends on the effectiveness of coordinated efforts that have evolved from the strategic planning level.

The main objective of the infection control effort is accomplished at the microlevel using the principles of educating, implementing, surveying, monitoring, and reporting the infection control processes. These principles are enacted by establishing and monitoring individual infection control practices among providers and the population being helped. The principles are applied proactively through a combination of clinical, managerial, and logistical planning, all of which are being assessed at the strategic level.

Best practices from after-action reports of major disasters should be compiled, analyzed, and published so the information is disseminated to individuals entrusted with infection control management and disaster response at all levels. For instance, "the main lesson learned from the severe acute respiratory syndrome (SARS) outbreak (of 2003) was that it was contained through the conscientious application of enhanced infection control measures at the national and local levels... Control of an emerging infection requires swift action by health care providers and an adequate public health infrastructure."[9]

A successful infection control program in disaster situations requires enormous planning efforts; dedicated, detail-oriented health care workers; and helpful tools including checklists that emphasize the basics of education, monitoring, surveillance, and reporting. Understanding the successes and failures of past disasters, while rehearsing how to react in a crisis today, will allow ordinary people to accomplish extraordinary things in the area of infection control and prevention.

ACKNOWLEDGMENTS

The authors thank US Army nurses Lieutenant Colonel Kim Smith and Major Yvonne Heib for their deployment wisdom, and Fluryanne Leach RN, chief of infection control and epidemiology service at Walter Reed Army Medical Center, for sharing her infection control wisdom.

REFERENCES

1. Toole MJ, Waldman RJ. The public health aspects of complex emergencies and refugee situations. Annu Rev Public Health 1997;18:283–312.
2. Murray CK, Hinkle MK, Yun HC. History of infections associated with combat-related injuries. J Trauma 2008;64(3):S221–31.
3. Western and Central Europe Chronology: the Black Death 1347–1351. Available at: http://www.thenagain.info/WebChron/westeurope/BlackDeath.html. Accessed July 5, 2009.
4. Cohen IB. Florence Nightingale. Available at: http://www.unc.edu/~nielsen/soci708/cdocs/cohen.htm. Accessed June 23, 2009.
5. Pierce JW, Writer JV. Yellow jack—how yellow fever ravaged America and Walter Reed discovered its deadly secrets. Hoboken (NJ): John Wiley & Sons, Inc; 2005.
6. Centers for Disease Control and Prevention. The Panama Canal. Available at: http://www.cdc.gov/malaria/history/panama_canal.htm. Accessed July 5, 2009.
7. History Learning Site. Poison Gas and World War One. Available at: http://www.historylearningsite.co.uk/poison_gas_and_world_war_one.htm. Accessed July 5, 2009.

8. Human Virology at Stanford. The Influenza Pandemic of 1918. Available at: http://virus.stanford.edu/uda. Accessed July 5, 2009.
9. Goldrick BA. The practice of infection control and applied epidemiology: a historical perspective. Am J Infect Control 2005;33(9):493–500.
10. Roup B, Kelley PW. Principles of infection control and prevention during military deployment. Textbooks of Military Medicine. Washington, DC: Borden Institute; 2005. p. 1251.
11. Mogadishu Somalia. Available at: http://www.usatoday.com/weather/climate/africa/somalia/wmogadis.htm; 2002. Accessed July 5, 2009.
12. Novel Swine-Origin Influenza A (H1N1) Virus Investigation Team, Dawood FS, Jain S, Finelli L, et al. Emergence of a novel swine-origin influenza A (H1N1) virus in humans. N Engl J Med 2009;360(25):2605–15.
13. Gostin LO, Bayer R, Fairchild AL, et al. Ethical and legal challenges posed by severe acute respiratory syndrome: implications for the control of severe infectious disease threats. JAMA 2003;290:3229–37.
14. Lubroth J, Morzaria S, Thiermann AB. Global strategy for highly pathogenic avian influenza: progressive control and eradication and postoutbreak recovery. In: Swayne DE, editor. Avian Influenza. Ames (IA): Blackwell Publishing; 2008. p. 561.
15. Knapp MB, McIntyre R, Sinkowitz-Cochran RL, et al. Assessment of health care personnel needs for training in infection control: one size does not fit all. Am J Infect Control 2008;36(10):757–60.
16. Izenberg S. Civilian application of military resources. Surg Clin North Am 2006;86(3):665–73.
17. Hayes AB, Weiser TG, Berry WR, et al. A surgical safety checklist to reduce morbidity and mortality in a global population. N Engl J Med 2009;360:491–9.
18. A Guidance for United Nations Field High Commissioner for Refugees Field Operations on Water and Sanitation Services. Field Guidance Manual. 2008. p. 5. Available at: http://www.unhcr.org/cgi-bin/texis/vtx/search?page=search&docid=49d080df2&query=water. Accessed March 24, 2010.
19. Lucci EB. Civilian preparedness and counter-terrorism: conventional weapons. Surg Clin North Am 2006;86(3):593.

Caring for Burn Patients at the United States Institute of Surgical Research: The Nurses' Multifaceted Roles

Maria Serio-Melvin, MSN, RN[a], Linda H. Yoder, PhD, MBA, RN[b,*],
Kathryn M. Gaylord, PhD, RN[a]

KEYWORDS

• Burns • Nursing care • Outcomes research • Military

The Burn Center is part of the US Army Institute of Surgical Research (USAISR), located within the Army's only level I trauma center, San Antonio Military Medical Center (SAMMC), formerly known as Brooke Army Medical Center in San Antonio, Texas. The USAISR, originally named the Surgical Research Unit, was established in 1943 to evaluate the role of newly discovered antibiotics in the treatment of war wounds. The unit was located at Halloran General Hospital, Staten Island, New York. In 1947 the Institute became a permanent unit and moved to Brooke General Hospital, at Fort Sam Houston, San Antonio, Texas.[1,2] In addition to studying antibiotics, the unit also was charged with investigating innovative surgical techniques and developments. In 1949, because of concern about the large number of possible casualties generated by nuclear weapons, the unit's mission expanded to encompass the study of thermal injuries. The implementation of improved grafting procedures and use of antibiotics in new applications grew along with this mission. Over the next decade, research was conducted to evaluate the use of plasma extenders, grafting, and preservation of blood vessels, and the use of an "artificial kidney."[2] In 1970 the Surgical Research Center was renamed the USAISR, acknowledging the daily balance between clinical care and research within the unit.[1]

The opinions or assertions contained herein are solely the views of the authors and should not be construed as official or reflecting the views of the Department of Defense or the United States Government.

[a] United States Army Institute of Surgical Research, Fort Sam Houston, Texas 78234, USA
[b] University of Texas at Austin School of Nursing, 1700 Red River, Austin, TX 78701, USA
* Corresponding author.
E-mail address: lyoder@mail.nur.utexas.edu

Nurs Clin N Am 45 (2010) 233–248
doi:10.1016/j.cnur.2010.02.001
0029-6465/10/$ – see front matter © 2010 Elsevier Inc. All rights reserved.

Today, the USAISR provides a full spectrum of burn services to the Department of Defense (DoD) and military service members from the point of injury to full recovery, which may be years later. The Burn Center averages between 400 and 500 annual admissions, approximately double the number of admissions to the other 124 American Burn Association (ABA)–verified civilian burn centers.[3] Since 2003, more than 800 United States Service members have been admitted for treatment of severe burn injuries, with an overall mortality rate of 5%.[4] Comprehensive, multidisciplinary care is provided by a staff consisting of more than 350 military and civil service federal employees and contract staff, in concert with consultants and ancillary services from SAMMC.

The USAISR's vision is to "integrate combat casualty care research missions/functions into a multi-faceted synergistic research capability with a clinical foundation and to sustain the DoD's world class adult burn center and lead the world in burn care research".[5] To achieve this vision, the Burn Center has a multifaceted mission. Staff provide (1) combat casualty care and products for injured soldiers, from self-aid through definitive care across the full spectrum of military operations; (2) state-of-the-art burn, trauma, and critical care to DoD beneficiaries around the world and civilians in the Brooke Army Medical Center trauma region; and (3) Burn Special Medical Augmentation Response Teams (also known as "USAISR burn flight teams").

The Burn Center serves as a prototype for burn units nationally and internationally. In 1996, the research focus of the Center's mission changed from thermal injury to the full spectrum of combat casualty care. The unit has cared for burn casualties from every conflict since World War II to the present, including the 1983 bombing in Beirut and the 1994 Pope Air Force Base plane crash, and dozens of other medical emergencies.[2]

The USAISR currently serves as the sole burn referral center for all DoD beneficiaries. As an ABA-verified burn referral center, it has a dual mission: caring for both burn casualties from the combat zone and civilian emergency burn victims, aged 17 years and older, in the Southwest Texas trauma region.[5,6] Referral criteria from the ABA state that critically burned patients are to be stabilized and transferred to a burn center. Examples of burns that meet referral criteria are[7]

1. Partial-thickness burns of greater than 10% of the total body surface area
2. Burns that involve the face, hands, feet, genitalia, perineum, or major joints
3. Third-degree burns in any age group
4. Electrical burns, including lightning injury
5. Chemical burns
6. Inhalation injury
7. Burn injury in patients with pre-existing medical disorders that could complicate management, prolong recovery, or affect mortality
8. Any patients with burns and concomitant trauma, such as fractures, in which the burn injury poses the greatest risk of morbidity or mortality
9. Burn injury in patients who require special social, emotional, or rehabilitative intervention.

CAUSES OF BURN INJURIES

According to the 2007 ABA National Burn Repository Report, common mechanisms of burn injuries among civilian patients are fire or flame (40% cases); scalding (30%); contact with a hot object (8%); electrical burns (4%); and chemical burns (3%). In that report, 43% of burns occurred in the home, 17% on the street or highway, and

8% at work; 32% were classified as "other."[3] Typically, at least 50% of the patients admitted to burn centers are critically burned as a result of ingesting alcoholic beverages.[8,9]

By contrast, individuals who are burned during combat most commonly sustain significant flame injuries along with polytrauma from injuries caused by conflicts with the enemy or in military training accidents.[10,11] For example, the typical cause of injury for combat casualties involves a military vehicle driving over an improvised explosive device (IED). These vehicles may transport four or more service members at any given time. When a vehicle encounters an IED, some of the service members survive and some may be killed by the explosion. For example, the distribution of injuries after an IED explosion could match the following scenario: one casualty walks away with hand and arm burns; another casualty sustains burns over 15% of his body, has a broken femur, and closed head injury; a third casualty has burns over 60% of his body with an inhalation injury, a broken arm, broken pelvis, broken right femur, and both feet mangled and eventually requiring amputation; the remaining crew members sustain minor or no injuries and are able to call for air evacuation and administer first aid.

In a recent study of patients burned while serving in Iraq, Injury Severity Scores were higher in combat casualties than in civilians.[11] This difference in severity scores was associated with a greater incidence of inhalation injury, larger body surface areas of full-thickness burn, more hand and face burns, penetrating abdominal injuries, and long-bone fractures. No significant differences were found, however, in overall mortality rates between civilian and military burn patients treated in the same burn center.

EXPORTING BURN CARE EXPERTISE

In 2003, after the start of Operation Iraqi Freedom, it was quickly realized that most medical personnel being sent to combat zones (ie, deploying medical personnel) did not know how to care for burn patients. Additionally, it became clear that advanced burn life support did not address the unique challenges that deploying medical personnel faced in combat zones. A team at the Army's Burn Center developed a combat burn life support course to augment the advanced burn life support course. These two courses were given in the continental United States, Germany, and the Middle East to over 1000 people in 2003 alone.[12] Currently, the staff at the USAISR, many of whom are bedside nurses, continue to conduct several different training forums to educate deploying military service members from all military services in both active and reserve status.

Since 2003, the USAISR education department has increased the number of personnel fourfold to coordinate training at various civilian venues and to meet the additional workload demands. In February 2008, a formalized clinical practicum was developed for military registered nurses (RNs), licensed practical nurses (LPNs), and military medics—enlisted service members with health care training largely focused on caring for battlefield injuries. This course is also available to other members of the health care team, such as physicians or other allied health care personnel. Every nursing staff member at the USAISR participates in the practicum by serving as a preceptor. The practicum allows for hands-on burn care experience before deployment. In 2008, seven different deploying units, comprised of 49 individuals (RNs, LPNs, operating room technicians, physicians, and medics) were trained for a combined total of 2390 clinical hours. On their departure, they each received a CD-ROM that contained burn care PowerPoint presentations, clinical practice guidelines, and a burn resuscitation flow sheet (Major Barry Rainwater, MA, RN, USAISR, Fort Sam Houston, TX, personal communication, May 2009). As a result of advances in Internet-based technology, deployed health care personnel also can obtain burn consultation services on the USAISR Web site.[13]

ABA-verified burn centers are expected to provide outreach burn care and prevention education to individuals living in the geographic area serviced. Staff at the Burn Center frequently teach civilian audiences about burn care and burn prevention at health fairs, high schools, universities, and professional conferences.

TRANSPORTING COMBAT CASUALTIES

Helicopter air evacuation capability is a key element to getting critically burned casualties to a hospital facility. The air evacuation helicopters that transport combat casualties are staffed with critical care or emergency department nurses from the Army Nurse Corps.[14] A burn surgeon is located at a combat support hospital (CSH) in Iraq, thereby bringing medical expertise in burn care directly to the battlefield. A CSH is an Army hospital located on the battlefield to provide hospitalization for up to 248 patients in all classes of care.[14] The actual numbers of beds, operating rooms, and personnel vary significantly according to workload. The multidisciplinary staff is similar to a level II trauma center in the United States, comprising an emergency department; an operating room; certified critical care and medical-surgical nurses; registered nurse anesthetists; anesthesiologists; and general and specialty surgeons (eg, orthopedic, cardiothoracic, vascular, and oral maxillofacial). Some CSHs also have a neurosurgeon on staff. The CSH also provides ancillary services, such as radiology, laboratory, pharmacy, ophthalmology, dermatology, dental, physical and occupational therapy, and nutrition care. With these capabilities, definitive care is provided to Wounded Warriors until they are stabilized for air evacuation to a regional medical center (Major John J. Melvin, MSN, RN, personal communication, June 2009).

The US Air Force provides air evacuation teams called Critical Care Air Transport Teams (CCATT) that consist of critical care physicians, nurses, and respiratory therapists.[15] One of the CCATT's responsibilities is to fly critically injured burned combat casualties from Iraq or Afghanistan to Landstuhl Regional Medical Center, Germany. Depending on the extent of the patient's burn injury, the CCATT may ultimately transport the patient from Germany to San Antonio. For severely burned patients, especially those with inhalation injuries, the Burn Special Medical Augmentation Response Team, also known as the "burn flight team," flies from San Antonio to Landstuhl and transports the patients to the Army Burn Center.[16]

THE BURN FLIGHT TEAM

The burn flight team comprises active duty health care personnel whose primary responsibility is to staff the burn intensive care unit (BICU). Service on the burn flight is an additional military duty. The team was created in 1953 and has transported over 2500 severely burned patients involved in catastrophes worldwide. Its mission is "to prepare for rapid worldwide deployment to evaluate, stabilize and transfer critically ill patients including severely burned and multiple trauma patients in an austere and ever-changing environment to the USAISR."[17] Rapid response is expected, requiring advanced preparation and personal sacrifice for members of the team and other BICU staff. When the team is called for a mission, it is for an undetermined length of time. This situation requires significant changes to the BICU schedule to fill staffing gaps. The burn flight team consists of a surgeon, a certified critical care registered nurse, an LPN, a respiratory therapist, and two enlisted soldiers, who are responsible for addressing all administrative and logistical issues regarding the flight team and the patients. All clinicians on the flight team need to demonstrate advanced clinical competence and have a minimum of 1 year of BICU experience.

Most commonly, the burn flight team deploys to Landstuhl Regional Medical Center. Once there, they continue efforts to stabilize the patients who are then flown more than 5000 miles across the Atlantic Ocean in the rear of a C-17 Globemaster III Air Force aircraft to the USAISR. This plane, which is a military version of a DC-9 aircraft, is designed to accommodate patients and equipped to give the same standard of care to the patients while in the air that is provided in the BICU in San Antonio. The flight time for such a mission is approximately 13 hours. To prepare for a mission, the RN, LPN, and respiratory therapist must anticipate the needs of the patients and ensure all necessary equipment and supplies are available. In-flight care requires 70-lb supply cases, a minimum of 11 per patient.

Outstanding clinical expertise and vigilance on behalf of all members of the team are essential to the burn flight team's success.[18] All burn flight team members attend a 2-week Air Force Critical Care Air Transport Team course that entails compression chamber training; medical and aircraft equipment awareness; emergency procedures in case of sudden decompression; physiologic changes caused by altitude, acceleration, and deceleration forces; and other hazards of flight. This training is important because the environmental conditions of flight influence the plan of care.[19]

A typical plan of care in flight includes (1) protecting and maintaining the airway; (2) ensuring ventilation and gas exchange; (3) maintaining hemodynamic stability by preventing shock; (4) preventing hypothermia; (5) preventing injury secondary to equipment dislodgement, falls, and immobility; and (6) preventing and monitoring for physiologic changes caused by altitude, such as gas expansion, hypoxia, and other hazards of flight. Provision of this level of nursing care is extremely difficult because the nurses' access to the patient is significantly hampered by the life-sustaining equipment attached to the canvas litters on which the patients are typically transported. Temperature control in the back of a transport aircraft is next to impossible, and patients are bundled in several special heat-conserving blankets to prevent hypothermia.[20] Additionally, poor lighting and diminished hearing caused by engine noise make caring for the patients extremely challenging.

CLINICAL OPERATIONS

At the USAISR, the entire spectrum of care (from intensive care to outpatient services) is provided to patients with burn injuries. The Burn Center has a 16-bed BICU, a dedicated operating room located next to the BICU, a 24-bed progressive care unit (PCU), and a burn clinic. For burn survivors, a rough estimate of the average length of hospital stay is slightly longer than 1 day per percentage point of total body surface area (TBSA) burned.[8] For patients with burns and polytrauma, however, the length of stay may be longer because of additional physical and psychological issues that require inpatient management. Furthermore, military service members may require and can seek outpatient burn wound care and rehabilitative services for years.

A large multidisciplinary team, led by the medical intensivist, holds bedside rounds every morning on each patient. Rounds last 1 to 2 hours depending on the number of patients and their acuity. The medical resident presents the patients by using a review of systems based on the medical model. At the end of each presentation, the intensivist asks all members of the team if there are any questions or concerns. Everyone attending rounds is encouraged to share pertinent information with the team. The team consists of attending burn surgeons and intensivists, physicians' assistants

(PAs), physicians in burn fellowships, medical residents, various types of health care students, a physical medicine and rehabilitation physician, reconstructive surgeons, a clinical dietician, behavioral medicine staff, social workers, and nurse case managers. The team also includes respiratory, physical, and occupational therapists and numerous RNs, such as the burn program manager, an infection control nurse, the Burn Center clinical nurse specialist (CNS), research RNs, the wound care coordinator, a charge nurse, the bedside RN, members from the nursing leadership team, and various consultants. After receiving feedback from the multidisciplinary team, the medical intensivist in collaboration with the attending burn surgeon makes final decisions about the plan of care. Unlike several other burn units, the Army Burn Center has behavioral medicine, respiratory therapy, and an inpatient and outpatient rehabilitation staff that exclusively care for burn patients.

There are over 120 nursing personnel employed in the Burn Center: 30% are military nurses and 70% are civilian nurses, with 20% of these being members of the civil service and 50% being agency nurses. At least 30% of the nursing staff is educated at the baccalaureate level, and several nurses have earned certifications in their specialty field. All members of the RN burn unit leadership have a master's degree. All the members of the nursing staff work synergistically to support the dual mission of clinical care and research. To work in the USAISR, a minimum of 1 year's experience in a nursing area, such as intensive care, the operating room, medical or surgical, or outpatient care, is required. The burn nursing experience among the nurses at the Burn Center ranges from weeks to 20 years (Colonel Kimberly K. Smith, MSN, RN, Fort Sam Houston, TX, personal communication, May 2009).

BURN INTENSIVE CARE UNIT

Nurses in the BICU provide care for patients with severe burns over 20% of their body, inhalation injuries, and circumferential extremity burns. These critical patients typically have significant polytrauma or comorbidities, hemodynamic instability, toxic epidermal necrotizing syndrome, necrotizing fasciitis, and other trauma for which the Burn Center is optimally designed. Using the American Association of Critical Care Nurses' synergy model[21] to describe typical burn patients, one would say they are moderately resilient, highly vulnerable, minimally stable, highly complex with moderate resources, do not participate in care, have moderate participation in decision making, and their hospital course is moderately predictable. Using this model, a typical patient on admission and for several weeks postburn would receive a score of 13 out of 40 points, where a low score indicates the criticality of the patient.[21]

Because of the criticality and high acuity of these patients, the nurse-staffing model is 1.5 nurses per patient. An RN is directly assigned to each patient and an LPN assists two RNs with their patients, especially to help with the hours of burn wound care that must be provided. The critical care nurses at the bedside must be extremely knowledgeable and skillful in burn wound care. In addition, they must also be responsible for continuous and vigilant monitoring of patients with the use of various forms of technology, such as the following (**Fig. 1**):

1. Cardiac monitors with four pressure waveforms that measure a minimum of central venous pressure and arterial blood pressure
2. Continuous cardiac output monitors
3. Ventilators
4. End-tidal carbon dioxide monitors
5. Intracranial pressure monitors

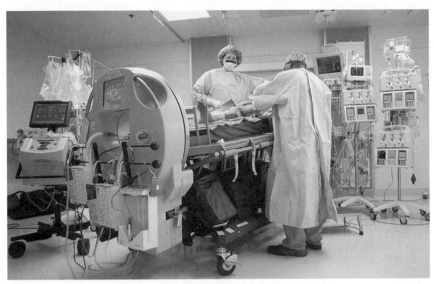

Fig. 1. A registered nurse and a licensed practical nurse in the burn intensive care unit use advanced technology to care for a critically burned soldier.

6. Continuous renal replacement therapy machines
7. Rotating specialty beds
8. Multiple intravenous pumps
9. Computer-assisted decision support computer programs that assist with glucose control, insulin drip rates, and burn fluid resuscitation
10. Glucose point-of-care testing machines
11. Electronic (computerized) medical records
12. A urimeter that measures hourly urine outputs and patients' core temperatures
13. Chest tubes.

Burn wound care involves dressing changes, applying various topical antimicrobial agents, and using hydrotherapy, all accomplished in environmental temperatures of 90°F to 100°F with 40% humidity because burn patients have difficulty maintaining their body temperature.[1] Personal protective equipment must always be worn during wound care, making the patient care environment extremely warm for the nurses.

CONTINUOUS RENAL REPLACEMENT THERAPY

Because of the nature of their injuries, burn patients are at high risk for infection, multi-system organ failure, and severe sepsis. In 2005, a continuous renal replacement therapy (CRRT) program was developed by the BICU's medical intensivist, the Burn Center's CNS, and experienced ICU nurses to provide another treatment for patients experiencing acute kidney injury. CRRT consists of using a machine to support kidney function, similar to dialysis, 24 hours a day. After the patient's kidney function and clinical signs and symptoms improve, the therapy is discontinued. Patients can be on this therapy from several hours to several months.[22–24]

CRRT has become the USAISR's standard treatment, particularly for patients who have septic shock with Acute Kidney Injury Network stage 2 (urinary output <0.5 mL/kg for 12 hours, double or triple baseline creatinine).[22–24] CRRT requires a physician's order and numerous nursing resources. When a patient needs CRRT, either one nurse is assigned to operate the CRRT machine and one or two other nurses care for the patient, or two nurses who know how to manage the CRRT machine are both assigned to care for the patient.

The nurses must be very knowledgeable about the principles of CRRT to understand and implement the plan of care for a patient on CRRT. Additionally, the nurse must do the following (Kellie Miller, BSN, RN, ISR CCRT Instructor, Fort Sam Houston, TX, personal communication, May 2009):

1. Understand how the CRRT system components work
2. Troubleshoot alarms
3. Set up and disassemble the CRRT machine
4. Monitor the CRRT system and its effect on the patient's status
5. Titrate anticoagulation medications based on laboratory values
6. Monitor filter appearance and longevity
7. Monitor electrolytes and the acid-base balance
8. Notify the physician of the patient's condition
9. Document all assessments and interventions.

Every 3 months, BICU CRRT nurses instruct other ICU RNs and LPNs about CRRT. The class consists of a 6-hour didactic component followed by 2 hours of hands-on practice. The nurses must then manage CRRT on three patients with a preceptor before they are considered completely trained. Approximately 50% of all BICU nurses are trained on this therapy with approximately 10 of the unit's nurses considered to be superusers. A superuser is scheduled to work on every shift to ensure a CRRT-trained nurse is always available. This program has been very successful to date. In burn patients diagnosed with acute renal injury, the Burn Center's in-hospital mortality rate is 62% compared with 86% in patients who did not receive this therapy.[22]

ICU WOUND CARE COORDINATOR

Because of the increased number of burn cases caused by combat operations, a wound care coordinator was hired. This coordinator, who trained with the burn surgeons and is extremely knowledgeable about burn wound care, has been instrumental in improving continuity of wound care, decreasing donor site infection rates, and decreasing pressure ulcers. Serving as an expert in burn wound care and negative pressure wound therapy, the wound care coordinator teaches or reinforces the principles of burn wound care during formal lectures and at the bedside to all personnel who work in the USAISR. The wound care coordinator also serves as a resource person, teacher, and consultant for SAMMC and the local civilian health care community.

OPERATING ROOM

Anecdotal estimates indicate that for every 10% TBSA of full-thickness burn, one surgery is required (Lieutenant Colonel [Retired] Edwin Alberto, MSN, RN, Fort Sam Houston, TX, personal communication, May 2009). The burn operating room is staffed with personnel exclusively assigned to this unit; they are available 24 hours per day 7 days per week to ensure dedicated support for burn casualties. The USAISR's two operating rooms supported more than 765 surgeries in 2008, all related to caring for patients with burns. ICU nurses provide postanesthesia care in the BICU. At times, trained nurses from the PCU may recover postoperative patients who went to the operating room directly from the PCU.

PROGRESSIVE CARE UNIT

Nurses in the 24-bed PCU provide care for patients transferred from the BICU, and patients admitted from the emergency department, burn clinic, CCATT, or burn flight team. Criteria for admission to this unit are that the patient must have open burn wounds over less than 20% TBSA, and the patient's cardiovascular and pulmonary systems must be stable. The two main goals of care in the PCU are to continue to assist the patient with recovery, focusing on the wound healing aspects of care, and to prepare the patient and family for discharge, focusing more on the emotional and psychological aspects of care. There is a patient educational component to both of these goals.

The PCU nurse must remain vigilant as the burn patient is recovering because these patients may have a large amount of open skin, thereby increasing their chances of electrolyte imbalance and hemodynamic instability caused by infection and sepsis. To facilitate burn wound healing, the patients continue with ongoing burn wound care, including intensive hydrotherapy; application of topical antibiotic creams, solutions, or dressings; and additional excision and grafting surgeries. Intravenous and oral antibiotics are commonly ordered.

Burn patients are in a hypermetabolic state and require high-protein, high-carbohydrate foods and beverages at all times. Part of the plan of care is to ensure that patients receive their daily nutritional requirements. The nurses must document calorie counts, administer several vitamins, and encourage patients to eat and drink nutritionally dense foods and beverages. This goal is very difficult to accomplish because these patients are thirsty but not hungry, making it imperative that everything ingested contributes to their daily caloric requirements. Milk, nutritional supplements, and foods high in vitamins and minerals are given to the patients. In the Burn Center it is rare for thermally injured patients to be allowed to drink water, Kool-Aid, or beverages containing caffeine or carbonation. These restrictions are required because those fluid sources tend to (1) drop the patients' sodium levels, (2) provide empty calories, and (3) keep patients from feeling hungry and eating healthy foods. The acuity of these patients is less than that of the patients in the BICU, but they continue to have a huge demand for wound care and they need considerable assistance with activities of daily living.

According to the synergy model, this type of patient could be classified as moderately resilient, moderately vulnerable, moderately stable, or moderately complex, with moderate resources, a moderate level of participation in care and decision making, and moderately predictable, for a total score of 24 out of 40 points.[21] The nurse-to-patient ratio is one nurse for two or three patients during the day and one nurse for three or four patients at night.

To prepare the patient for discharge, the nurses address self-image issues related to disfigurement caused by the burn injury and, in some cases, amputations resulting from polytrauma. The PCU nurses also work closely with the rehabilitation staff to increase patients' independence with activities of daily living, transfers, and ambulation. Although extensive painful burn wound care is still needed, the nurses work with the patients to decrease the amount of narcotics and benzodiazepines they need, while continuing to provide adequate pain and anxiety management. Another goal is to encourage the patient to become less dependent on family members for decision making. As soon as the patients are medically capable of making independent decisions, a gradual process is initiated so that patients start making decisions about their medical care, ongoing financial issues, and family dynamics. Military service members who learn they can no longer remain in the military because of the extent of their injuries are encouraged to start planning for future occupations and deciding on the location of their future home. Efforts also are made to prepare the patient and family for community and family reintegration and eventual discharge home.

For burned military service members and civilian emergency patients, the main requirements used to determine if a patient meets USAISR discharge criteria are the amount and intensity of burn wound care; independence with activities of daily living; the ability to stand, transfer, or ambulate; pain controlled with oral medications; appropriate decision making; and stable mental status. Military service members who do not reside in the San Antonio, Texas, area may be discharged "home" to The Fisher House, which is similar to a Ronald McDonald House for patients and their families. Patients and families may also reside in a military hotel. The four Fisher Houses and the hotel are located across the street from the hospital, making access to care and attending outpatient follow-up appointments much easier for patients and families. During this transition period, the patient's care is provided by family members and friends, who may have left their homes and jobs in other parts of the country for an indefinite time to provide physical care and emotional support to the burned service member.

BURN CLINIC

For military service members and some civilian patients, the USAISR provides continuing outpatient burn wound care and rehabilitation services during regular clinic hours, Monday through Friday. This care may include measurement for compression garments and outpatient reconstructive surgery services in the Burn Clinic. Similar to their inpatient stays, the patients in the Burn Clinic receive care from a multidisciplinary team. Patients may need the kind of care provided in the Burn Clinic for years, but this need gradually diminishes as the patients become healthier over time. The Burn Clinic is staffed by attending burn surgeons, two PAs, an RN, three LPNs, a physical or occupational therapist, and a medical clerk. A reconstructive surgeon, physical medicine and rehabilitation physicians, and a person who measures the patients for compression garments also are available as needed. Behavioral medicine, chaplain, and dietician staff members quickly respond to requests for their assistance.

PAs, in collaboration with the attending surgeon, are responsible for the medical management of patients in the Burn Clinic. The RN is the nurse manager of the clinic and develops the nursing and educational plan of care on all patients. The RN also ensures that the clinic functions smoothly and any problems that may arise are quickly resolved. The LPNs do most of the dressing changes and contribute to the nursing plan of care. The LPNs educate patients and family members as needed to support the plan of care. A therapist helps the patients with both physical and occupational therapy needs. Because these patients are followed for such a long time, it is common that unique relationships are formed with members of the Burn Clinic team. The Burn Clinic staff handled over 5800 visits in 2008.

For military personnel who have sustained burn injuries, the goal is to continue to care for all of their injuries within the military system. If the patient wants to stay in the military, the military community will do everything within its capabilities to ensure that goal is met. A "triad of care" has been established for each wounded warrior.[25] This triad consists of (1) the primary care manager, who is the service member's primary doctor or nurse practitioner; (2) the patient's case manager, usually an RN, who coordinates all health care appointments and ensures continuity of care for all injuries; and (3) an enlisted liaison who ensures the warrior's and family's basic needs are met. A Warrior Family Support Center also is available and provides a vast array of resources to assist the patient and family with adjustment to their new state of "normal."

OTHER NURSING ROLES

Nurses hold several other nursing roles within the USAISR. Each of these roles directly or indirectly influences patient care and ultimately improves outcomes. They are summarized next.

Clinical Nurse Specialist

The Burn Center CNS is a master's degree–prepared critical care nurse who has extensive knowledge and experience in burn nursing from the point of injury in the combat zone through air evacuation, critical care, progressive care, and lengthy outpatient follow-up care. The CNS is an advanced practice nurse who functions as a clinical expert, educator, consultant, and researcher focused on the care of burn patients. Incorporated within each of these functions, the CNS is a role model, patient-family advocate, change agent, resource manager, facilitator of ethical decisions, and leader.[26] As a clinical expert, in collaboration with the multidisciplinary staff, the CNS monitors the clinical care of patients and gathers and disseminates evidence to improve clinical practice through process improvement initiatives and educational programs and consultation services.

As an educator, the CNS directly affects the USAISR competency, orientation, and predeployment programs, and several SAMMC educational programs, and participates in community outreach education initiatives. Burn care consists of very specialized skills possessed by few health care providers. The CNS provides consultative services for SAMMC; all the uniformed services; and civilian local, national, and international communities. This individual provides presentations about burn care at national and international conferences. The CNS also disseminates clinical findings from the USAISR research program by peer-reviewed manuscripts, abstracts, and posters. The CNS participates in interdisciplinary research by serving as an associate investigator on various physician-led studies and developing research studies from clinical questions that arise. A recently conducted study by a burn CNS investigated error rates in point-of-care glucometers among patients with anemia. As a result of that research, glucometer manufacturers were contacted and algorithms within the glucometers were corrected to account for anemia.[27]

Burn Program Manager

The burn program manager is a baccalaureate or master's degree–prepared RN who assists the USAISR leadership team with administrative functions within the Burn Center. This nurse ensures that all verification requirements dictated by the American College of Surgeons and the ABA are met for SAMMC to maintain its level I trauma center status and for the USAISR to retain its ABA Burn Center verification status. The burn program manager also assists the organization in meeting all requirements for Joint Commission accreditation and ensures that credentials of the medical staff are current.

To decrease errors and near misses, the burn program manager facilitates and monitors multidisciplinary process improvement initiatives. He or she then communicates findings to the SAMMC-USAISR health care staff and external agencies, such as transferring civilian facilities, military facilities in the combat area that transferred the patient to the Burn Center, and the Veteran's Administration health care team. This nurse also is responsible for collecting data and maintaining the National Burn Repository database, allowing the USAISR to share burn information with the rest of the world.[28]

Infection Control Practitioner

The infection control practitioner is an RN with a bachelor's degree and certification from the Certification Board of Infection Control and Epidemiology.[29] The infection control practitioner is responsible for infection prevention and infection control surveillance. This nurse develops, implements, and evaluates process improvement initiatives to decrease hospital-acquired infections in this high-risk, vulnerable patient population. She or he reports findings to the health care team in the Burn Center and directly to the executive leaders of the USAISR.

Research Nurses

Clinical research is an integral part of daily patient care within the USAISR. Research RNs counsel patients and families, invite them to participate in a variety of prospective and retrospective research studies, and obtain informed consent. Currently, research nurses facilitate approximately 15 different protocols. They also assist other study investigators in writing protocols, assessing the protocols to determine their impact on nursing practice and workload, and writing addendums to extant protocols. The research nurses collect data for several protocols at a time and are responsible for all administrative requirements as dictated by the SAMMC Investigational Review Board, the USAISR Office of Regulatory Compliance and Quality Management, and the US Army Medical Research and Material Command. The ongoing research mission within the USAISR has provided numerous burn care improvements to military and civilian health care.[27,30,31]

Nurses in Behavioral Medicine Roles

Coping with the physical and psychological issues associated with burn injuries on a continuing basis can be very difficult for patients, families, and the health care staff. A robust behavioral medicine team is available to address these complex psychosocial issues. A psychiatric mental health nurse practitioner provides clinical care to the patients, many of whom have psychiatric comorbidities, traumatic brain injury, post-traumatic stress disorder, acute stress disorder, or exhibit poor coping skills, all of which complicate recovery and require long-term follow-up. A psychiatric mental health CNS also is available to assist families with complex and very stressful issues.

Wounded warriors and some civilians, such as firefighters, are burned as a result of being in harm's way, serving their country. By virtue of sustaining severe burns and polytrauma, self-image, livelihood, and personal and professional relationships are often affected. Additionally, burn patients may have lost legs, arms, and possibly their eyesight. Many wounded warriors identify with their roles in the military. These service members typically were in excellent physical shape and served as the main financial provider for their families. Because of their severe injuries, wounded warriors have a higher risk for developing psychosocial problems, especially when having to rely on family members or friends to care for their basic needs, 24 hours a day, 7 days a week (Colonel Kathryn M. Gaylord, PhD, APRN, Fort Sam Houston, TX, personal communication, May 2009).[32]

Many of the military health care team members have deployed to a combat zone at least once during their military career and can identify with their patients, often resulting in the development of compassion fatigue. Also, because of the nature of burn care, there may be a high turnover rate among the military nursing staff.[33] A behavioral health team staffed with bachelor's and master's degree–prepared psychiatric nurses is available to assist the USAISR staff in dealing with the emotional toll of caring for the devastating injuries suffered by civilian and military burn patients. In addition, there is a respite room available in the Burn Center where caregivers can relax and get some relief from the stress of the day.[1]

NURSING-LED RESEARCH

Research at the USAISR includes animal research, bench science, and clinical research. Clinical research is conducted in the Burn Center by a multidisciplinary team that includes the CNS and a doctorally prepared nurse investigator. The CNS focuses on studies related to the clinical issues associated with burn treatment. The doctorally prepared nurse completes outcome studies that focus on psychological issues associated with burn injury. Such studies include research on quality of life, posttraumatic stress disorder, depression, mild traumatic brain injury, and pain (**Box 1**).

Box 1
Nursing research at the USAISR Burn Center

Clinical nurse-led research at USAISR Burn Center

Computer decision support to achieve glycemic control in the intensive care unit

Algorithmic adjustment to correct artificial elevation in point-of-care glucose measurement caused by nonoptimal hematocrit

Quantification of protein loss from negative pressure wound therapy in burn, trauma, and surgical patients

Psychosocial nurse-led research at USAISR Burn Center

Longitudinal outcomes from a military burn center

Longitudinal outcomes of burned service members treated at a military burn center

Longitudinal outcomes of burned civilians treated at a military burn center

Long-term outcomes in burned Operation Enduring Freedom/Operation Iraqi Freedom veterans

A comparison of posttraumatic stress disorder and mild traumatic brain injury in burned military service members

A comparison of posttraumatic stress disorder between combat casualties and civilians treated at a military burn center

Pain and sleep disturbance in soldiers with extremity trauma

The correlation between ketamine and posttraumatic stress disorder in burned service members

The effect of propranolol on posttraumatic stress disorder in burned service members

Effect of cranial electrical stimulation on pain in burned patients in an outpatient setting

A feasibility study using gradual virtual reality exposure therapy and D-cycloserine for treatment of combat-related posttraumatic stress disorder in burned service members

Enhancing prolonged exposure therapy with family education

Research concerning the quality of life of burn patients began at the USAISR in the late 1990s with a focus on describing how patients cope and adapt after discharge from the Burn Center. Collaborations with external organizations, such as the Veterans Administration, have been developed to identify issues surrounding the transition of care of wounded warriors from military to Veterans Administration health care settings. Wounded warriors and civilian burn patients are enrolled in most studies to examine differences and similarities between these two groups.

The USAISR Burn Center clinical staff members recognize that they have a critical role in research. They participate in research by providing clinical ideas or questions to investigators and acting as associate investigators on studies. Although patient care is their primary focus, participation in research provides an opportunity for staff members to take part in expanding the science regarding burn care.

SUMMARY

Providing nursing care to military and civilian burn patients admitted to the USAISR is challenging and rewarding. The complexity of assessment skills and care provision required is demanding, even for experienced clinicians. The military has a unique culture of "caring for our own." Simultaneously, the Army Burn Center offers a service to the civilian community through burn care provision and innovative research that decreases morbidity and mortality. The USAISR health care team has set burn care standards in the past through providing important fluid resuscitation formulas and delivering innovative nursing care in combat zones. The interdisciplinary team at the Burn Center continues to work diligently to increase survival of civilians and Wounded Warriors and attempts to maximize long-term quality of life for the patients and families they encounter.

REFERENCES

1. Vaughn D. Treating the wounds of war. Military officer 2009;June:54–7.
2. United States Army Institute of Surgical Research. Unit history. Available at: http://www.usaisr.amedd.army.mil/history.html. Accessed May 1, 2009.
3. American Burn Association. Resources factsheet. Available at: http://www.ameriburn.org/resources_factsheet.php. Accessed May 15, 2009.
4. Gomez R, Murray CK, Hospenthal DR, et al. Causes of mortality by autopsy findings of combat casualties and civilian patients admitted to a burn unit. J Am Coll Surg 2009;208(3):348–54.
5. United States Army Institute of Surgical Research. Organization vision/mission. Available at: http://www.usaisr.amedd.army.mil/mv.html. Accessed May 1, 2009.
6. American Burn Association. Burn center verification. Available at: http://www.ameriburn.org/verification_verifiedcenters.php. Accessed May 15, 2009.
7. American Burn Association. Burn center referral criteria. Available at: http://www.ameriburn.org/BurnCenterReferralCriteria.pdf?PHPSESSID=c29e8070a683410fd97a5756aaa6e53d. Accessed May 15, 2009.
8. Albright JM, Kovacs EJ, Gamelli RL, et al. Implications of formal alcohol screening in burn patients. J Burn Care Res 2009;30(1):62–91.
9. Silver GM, Albright JM, Schermer CR, et al. Adverse clinical outcomes associated with elevated blood alcohol levels at the time of burn injury. J Burn Care Res 2008;29(5):784–9.
10. Kauvar DS, Wolf SE, Wade CE, et al. Burns sustained in combat explosions in Operations Iraqi and Enduring Freedom (OIF/OEF explosion burns). Burns 2006;32(7):853–7.

11. Wolf SE, Kauvar DS, Wade CE, et al. Comparison between civilian burns and combat burns from Operation Iraqi Freedom and Operation Enduring Freedom. Ann Surg 2006;243(6):786–92.

12. Barillo DJ, Cancio LC, Hutton BG, et al. Combat burn life support: a military burn-education program. J Burn Care Rehabil 2005;26(2):162–5.

13. United States Army Institute of Surgical Research. Burn consultation services. Available at: http://www.usaisr.amedd.army.mil/contacts.html. Accessed May 15, 2009.

14. FM 4-02.01 Theater Hospitalization. Headquarters, Department of the Army. Washington, DC: Author; 2005.

15. Smith KK. Critical care nursing in an austere environment. Crit Care Med 2008; 36(Suppl 7):297–303.

16. Renz EM, Cancio LC, Barillo DJ, et al. Long range transport of war-related burn casualties. J Trauma 2008;64(Suppl 2):136–44.

17. Ross G, Stout LR, Renz E, et al. U.S. Army Burn Flight Team. Poster presented at the annual meeting of the American Burn Association. Chicago, IL, May 10–13; 2005.

18. Greely HL. Duty, honor, country. Advance for Nurses 5(24):13–6.

19. Topley DK, Schmelz J, Henkemius-Kirschbaum J, et al. Critical care nursing expertise during air transport. Mil Med 2003;168(10):822–6.

20. Bridges E, editor. Battlefield and disaster nursing pocket guide. Sudbury (MA): Jones & Bartlett; 2009. p. 87–90.

21. American Association of Critical Care Nurses. The AACN synergy model for patient care. Available at: http://www.aacn.org/WD/Certifications/Content/synmodel.pcms?mid=2869&menu#Patient. Accessed May 15, 2009.

22. Chung KK, Lundy JB, Matson JJ, et al. Continuous venovenous hemofiltration in severely burned patients with acute kidney injury: a cohort study [abstract]. Crit Care 2009;13(3):R62.

23. Chung KK, Perkins RM, Oliver JD III. Renal replacement therapy in support of combat operations. Crit Care Med 2008;36(Suppl 7):365–9.

24. Chung KK, Juncos LA, Wolf SE, et al. Continuous renal replacement therapy improves survival in severely burned military casualties with acute kidney injury. J Trauma 2008;64(Suppl 2):179–85.

25. Warrior Transition Office. U.S. army medical command warrior transition office concept of operations for warrior transition unit organizational inspection program. Falls Church (VA): Office of the Surgeon General of the Army; 2008.

26. Bell L, editor. Scope of practice and standards of professional performance for the acute and critical care clinical nurse specialist. Aliso Viejo (CA): American Association of Critical-Care Nurses; 2000. p. 8.

27. Mann EA, Salinas J, Pidcoke HF, et al. Error rates resulting from anemia can be corrected in multiple commonly used point-of-care glucometers. J Trauma 2008;64(1):15–20.

28. American College of Surgeons. Resources for optimal care of the injured patient. Available at: http://www.facs.org/trauma/resourcesoptimal.html; 2006. Revised July 30, 2007. Accessed May 15, 2009.

29. Certification Board of Infection Control and Epidemiology. Certification criteria for the infection control practitioner. Available at: http://www.cbic.org/. Accessed May 15, 2009.

30. Mann EA, Pidcoke HF, Salinas J, et al. The impact of intensive insulin protocols and restrictive blood transfusion strategies on glucose measurement in American

Burn Association (ABA) verified burn centers. J Burn Care Res 2008;29(5): 718–23.

31. Mann EA, Pidcoke HF, Salinas J, et al. Accuracy of glucometers should not be assumed [comment]. Am J Crit Care 2007;16(6):531–2.

32. Gaylord KM, Cooper DB, Mercado JM, et al. Incidence of posttraumatic stress disorder and mild traumatic brain injury in burned service members: preliminary report. J Trauma 2008;64(Suppl 4):200–5.

33. Gaylord KM, Smith KK, Blackbourne LH. Compassion fatigue: caring for the caregiver. Poster presented at the annual meeting of the American Burn Association. San Antonio (TX), March 24–27; 2009.

The Documentation of Pain Management During Aeromedical Evacuation Missions

Di Lamb, MA, BSc (Hons), PMRAFNS

KEYWORDS

- Pain-management documentation • Clinical-effectiveness audit
- Aeromedical evacuation • Clinical standards

Health care governance initiatives implemented by the Aeromedical Evacuation (AE) Squadron, based at Royal Air Force, Lyneham, United Kingdom, focus on quality and performance improvements via a program of clinical-effectiveness audit. Robust governance of clinical standards demands that operational procedures are regularly assessed to ensure patients continue to receive the best possible care during AE. Modern warfare has generated a significant increase in blast injuries over recent years,[1] which demand careful management during planning and while undertaking air transfer. Pain management following multiple injuries can be challenging even when a patient is cared for in a stationary health care setting; this is further complicated by the additional stressors of flight. Factors such as movement, a decreased partial pressure of oxygen at altitude, vibration, noise, immobility, and limited climate control can exacerbate a patient's experience of pain.[2,3] For this reason, pain management during aeromedical transfer was prioritized for review in the clinical effectiveness audit program.

The review of pain management was divided into a number of phases, which will be outlined in turn.

STUDY ONE
Aim

The aim of Study One was to investigate the AE Squadron Flight Nurses' (FNs') experiences of managing patients' pain during the aeromedical phase of transfer to a UK medical facility.

Aeromedical Evacuation Cell–OC PA/AELO, The Royal Centre for Defence Medicine, Selly Oak Hospital, Raddlebarn Road, Birmingham, B29 6JD, UK
E-mail address: Di.Lamb@uhb.nhs.uk

Nurs Clin N Am 45 (2010) 249–260
doi:10.1016/j.cnur.2010.02.012
0029-6465/10/$ – see front matter © 2010 Published by Elsevier Inc.

nursing.theclinics.com

Method

A questionnaire was distributed inviting all permanent AE Squadron FNs (n = 19), including three Registered Mental Nurses, to qualify and quantify any issues relating to patients' in-flight pain management (**Box 1**).

The dataset provided a cumulative knowledge base totaling 33 years, ranging from 4 months to 11 years, of recent experience within the AE specialty. Descriptive statistics were calculated for quantitative data and content analysis was performed on qualitative data to identify patterns or themes, which linked incidents and concepts. Subsequently, a coding schedule was constructed that was reviewed by a colleague, independent of the project, and discussed at length until agreement was reached in providing reliable themes.

Findings

A summary of quantitative data analysis is tabulated in **Table 1**.
Qualitative data is summarized in **Fig. 1**.

DISCUSSION

The findings of this audit suggest that permanent AE Squadron personnel do not regularly experience problems with the management of patients' pain in-flight and, of the two experiences highlighted, both related to inappropriate pain management regimes at the dispatching medical facility before departure from the emplaning airfield. One particular case identified inadequate communication by the Medical Liaison Officer with relevant medical practitioners before the FN's arrival at their location, despite

---

Box 1
In-flight pain management survey

Q1. Have you ever experienced an AE flight during which you felt unable to adequately control a patient's pain?

Q2. If you answered "Yes" to Q1, please give brief details of the patient's clinical condition and why you were unable to adequately control the pain.

Q3. Do you believe the environment in which the patient was being transported exacerbated the problems you experienced with their pain management?

Q4. If you answered "Yes" to Q3, please explain how the transportation environment exacerbated problems with pain management.

Q5. Do you feel limited when caring for patients in pain during a flight because you do not have a clearly defined pain algorithm to follow?

Q6. In your opinion, are the analgesic drugs you currently carry in the SKAI[a] bag adequate to treat pain experienced by your patient case mix?

Q7. If you answered "No" to Q6, please indicate what problems you have experienced with the currently available SKAI bag analgesic drugs.

Q8. In your opinion, on average when you do administer analgesia in-flight? Is it a result of a patient's request for pain control or your suggestion that pain control is clinically indicated?

Q9. Please outline ways in which you feel pain management for AE patients could be improved.

[a] The name given to the standard equipment bag carried by nursing personnel on AE flights.

| Table 1 |||
| **Quantitative data analysis** |||
Question	Yes	No
Q1. Have you ever experienced an AE flight during which you felt unable to adequately control a patient's pain?	13%	87%
Q5. Do you feel limited when caring for patients in pain during a flight because you do not have a clearly defined pain algorithm to follow?	27%	73%
Q6. In your opinion, are the analgesic drugs you currently carry in the SKAI (medical equipment) bag adequate to treat pain experienced by your patient casemix?	100%	—
Q8. In your opinion, on average when you do administer analgesia in-flight, it is as a result of:	The Patient's Request 27%	Clinical Indication 67% Both 6%

specific requests for prescriptions to be reviewed before flight. A more robust mechanism for personnel to address appropriate pain management strategies before the AE flight would be clearly beneficial. Aircraft scheduling, which is unfortunately prone to delays, often dictates the timescale of a patient's repatriation; thereby minimizing the time a FN has available to assess pain once on the ground. Therefore, overseas Medical Liaison personnel and Medical Officers have an essential role in ensuring pain management is effective before the AE escort's arrival and that medication and procedures are in place to maintain analgesia during all phases of transfer. A previously tested pharmacologic regime, together with adjuncts to manage the transfer

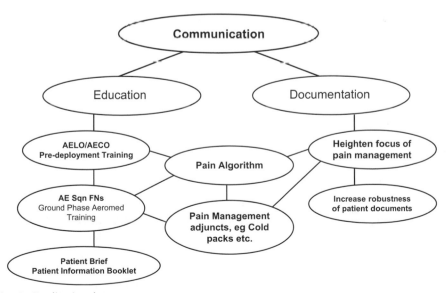

Fig. 1. Qualitative data summary.

environment, such as cold packs, pillows, and position are then more likely to effectively maintain adequate pain control. However, this system is dependant on appropriate training, which should raise awareness of the logistical limitations associated with the AE transfer environment and thereby ensure that in-flight pain is not regarded as the sole responsibility of the FN.

The qualitative data produced a number of themes suggesting pain management could be improved during AE. The overarching issue would appear to be communication, which could be further divided into education and documentation. Long-haul and short-haul care plans in use by the AE Squadron at that time did not utilize a standard pain score. During short-haul flights, a scale of 0 to 5 was used (0 = no pain, 2–3 = moderate pain, 5 = severe pain). During long-haul flights 0 to 5 and 0 to 10 pain score scales were used (0 = no pain, 5 = moderate pain, 10 = worst pain ever). This lack of consistency added unnecessary complication and it was recommended that an agreed standard for scoring pain irrespective of the length of flight sector should be introduced.

A pain assessment chart (**Fig. 2**) shown below, was proposed, approved, and implemented into standard AE documentation. This introduced a four-point pain score and complemented the scoring system used at the Royal Center for Defense Medicine in Birmingham, the Role 4 facility that receives British casualties.

All respondents reported that the drugs carried in their SKAI bags permitted them to adequately manage pain experienced by their patients. This suggested that the need for anything stronger than codeine, over and above that already prescribed by the dispatching medical facility, had not been experienced. The majority of respondents (67%) would administer analgesia when clinically indicated and 27% awaited it being requested by the patient. This further illustrated the need to raise pain management awareness and improve the associated documentation. However, it must be acknowledged that three potential respondents were psychiatric nurses whose patient case mix would be unlikely to experience physical pain; therefore, awaiting their patient's request for analgesia would be acceptable practice.

Three of the four respondents to Q5, who perceived their care of patients in pain to be limited by the lack of an algorithm, had been qualified for only 3 to 4 years. Therefore, a need was identified for the design and authorization of a management tool to benefit the more junior personnel. The approved algorithm is illustrated in **Figs. 2–4** as an interim measure to the implementation of Patient Group Directives (PGDs).

STUDY TWO
Aim

This study was undertaken concurrently with Study One to establish the completeness of pain management documentation during AE missions at that time.

Method

The audit was conducted in June 2007 by means of retrospective analysis of in-flight nursing and medical notes; it comprised 140 patients on strategic flights from all destinations and created a manageable dataset for the auditor.

Each flight file was scrutinized for the following data:

1. Date of transfer.
2. Flight details.
3. Dependency category of patient.
4. Description of patient illness or injuries.

White Copy – Patient's Notes
Orange Copy – Aeromed File

PROTECT - MEDICAL

FMed 1043
(Introduced February 2008)

PAIN ASSESSMENT CHART

Date: _____ Departing Airfield: _____ Flight Number: _____

Patient's Details

Service
Number: _____ Rank: _____

Name &
Inits: _____

Date of birth: _____ Unit: _____

Escorts Details

Service
Number: _____ Rank: _____

Name &
Inits: _____

1.   **Respiratory Rate:**   While patient is at rest count respiratory rate for one minute.

2.   **Sedation score:**   Look at the patient and decide which of the following apply:

Awake   0
Dozing intermittently   1
Mostly sleeping   2
Only awakens when roused 3

3.   **Pain assessment score:**   Ask the patient, "Which of the following words best describes
the   pain you are experiencing at the moment?"

No pain   0
Mild pain   1
Moderate pain   2
Severe pain   3

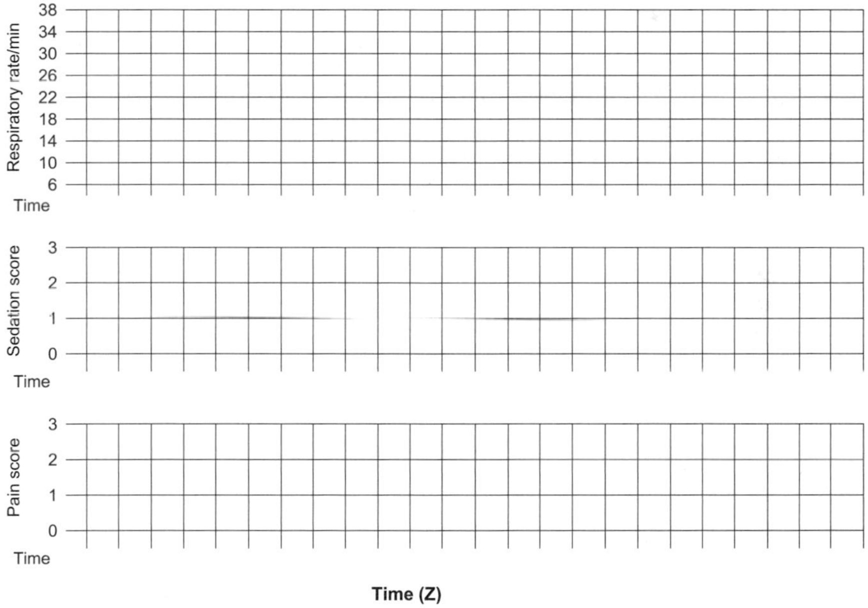

Fig. 2. Pain management chart.

5. Battle or non-battle injuries.
6. Analgesia regime.
7. Number of times a pain score was documented.
8. The level of the pain scores if documented.
9. Whether pain had been commented on in the narrative.

AEROMEDICAL EVACUATION SQUADRON

STANDARD OPERATING PROCEDURE   SOP 7.8.9

PAIN MANAGEMENT DOCUMENTATION

Reference:

A.   TMW/1250/15/AES dated 22 Nov 07.

AIM

1.   The aim of this SOP is to provide guidance to all members of the AE Squadron as to how a patient's pain should be managed and documented throughout an AE mission.

TASK IN OUTLINE

1.   Prior to departing Tactical Medical Wing, the Team Leader should speak to medical personnel at their destination to gain a comprehensive brief regarding the patient's current pain status and management regime. Due to minimal turn-around times at the destination airfield, this is vital in ensuring a patient's analgesia is appropriately prescribed and is available to the escort on arrival. Should specific analgesia be required this additional time will better facilitate it being obtained via Medical Logistics Flight. Any communication with personnel overseas should be documented in the patient's flight folder.

2.   During the patient's initial assessment by the escort following arrival at the enplaning airfield, the current analgesia regime should be checked to ensure it has been correctly prescribed and is sufficient to maintain pain control within tolerable limits for the duration of the AE mission. It must be appreciated that the patient will have been resting for a period of time prior to this assessment and it will be necessary to consider any additional discomfort generated as a direct result of their sudden movement or vibration from the aircraft.

3.   The Pain Management Algorithm overleaf will provide guidance to personnel when administering analgesia during an AE mission. Should there be any concerns regarding the escort's ability to control pain within the outlined parameters, the Medical Officer should be contacted, if available, and consideration given to reclassifying the patient unfit to fly. Discuss this with SO2 Aeromed at the Aeromedical Evacuation Control Centre at RAF Brize Norton if there are any outstanding concerns.

4.   Each time the patient's pain is assessed; a score should be documented in the flight folder. Should the patient require additional analgesia during the AE mission, this should be administered in accordance with the prescription chart and assessment of its efficiency one-hour later. Additional scores must be annotated in the flight folder.

5.   The flight folder is a legal document. In a court of law any omissions in care-related documentation suggests it did not happen. Robust documentation is therefore vital for practitioners to support their delivery of the highest standards of care.

TMW/1250/15/AES   Issue No 1

Issue Date: 1 Feb 08   Review Date: Nov 08

Fig. 3. Pain management algorithm.

Findings

Findings are presented in **Table 2**.

Discussion

The audit of AE paperwork identified that, of a dataset comprising a sample of 140 patients, 42% had no record of pain management in their notes despite 71% being

AEROMEDICAL EVACUATION SQUADRON
STANDARD OPERATING PROCEDURE   SOP 7.8.10

PAIN MANAGEMENT DOCUMENTATION

Algorithm to manage pain during an AE mission

Prior to departure from the UK:
- Make a request to the AELO/AECO for analgesia to be correctly prescribed for the duration of flight to the UK.
- Ensure non-standard SKAI bag drugs can be uplifted in the UK, at location or discuss alternatives and have them prescribed.

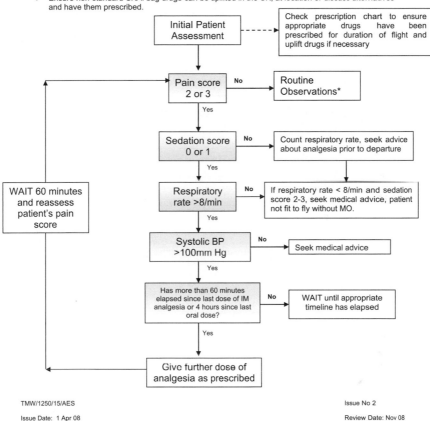

TMW/1250/15/AES   Issue No 2

Issue Date: 1 Apr 08   Review Date: Nov 08

Fig. 4. Pain management algorithm (continued). If pain score 1 and 4 to 6 hours have elapsed since last analgesia administration, consider a further oral dose as prescribed to prevent pain score escalating. (*Data from* Gould TH, Crosby DL, Harmer M, et al. Policy for controlling pain after surgery: effect of sequential changes in management. Br Med J 1992;305:1187–93.)

prescribed at least one type of analgesia. Conversely, 100% of Critical Care Air Support Team (CCAST) patients had their pain management well documented. A standard CCAST patient observation chart incorporates sedation and pain scoring with heart rate, pulse, blood pressure, and so forth, which are documented at least hourly; promoting it as the "fifth vital sign." This heightened profile of pain management is perhaps the prompt that was omitted from standard AE documentation at that time.

Table 2
Study two findings

Dependency[a] of Patient	4	3	2	1 Critical Care Air Support Team (CCAST)
Number audited	100	25	7	8

Dependency of Patient	4	3	2	1	Average
% of patients with recorded pain score	42	36	43	100	44

Ser	Question	June 2007 audit
1	Number of flight folders audited	140
2	Number of battle-injured patients	42
3	Percentage of patients prescribed at least one form of analgesia	71%
4	Percentage of patients with documented pain scores	44%
5	Percentage of patients with pain mentioned in the text but not scored	14%
6	Percentage of Battle Injured patients with documented pain assessment	54%
7	Percentage of Non-Battle Injured patients with documented pain assessment	36%
8	Number of patients with pain documented as ≤3 (0–10 scale)	46 (33%)
10	Number of patients with pain documented as > 3 (0–10 scale)	15 (11%)
12	Percentage of patients with no mention of pain management in their flight folder	42%

[a] Dependency 4 patients do not require nursing attention in flight but might need assistance with mobility or bodily functions. Dependency 3 patients are those that are not expected to deteriorate during flight but who require nursing or management of simple oxygen therapy, an intravenous infusion, or a urinary catheter. Dependency 2 patients, although not requiring intensive support, require regular, frequent monitoring and whose condition may deteriorate in flight. Such patients might include those who require management of a combination of oxygen administration, one or more intravenous infusions and multiple drains or catheters. Dependency 1 patients require intensive support during flight, such as mechanical ventilation, monitoring of central venous pressure or cardiac monitoring and may be unconscious or under general anesthesia.

However, worthy of note is that the very nature of a critically ill patient's clinical condition demands that pain and precise monitoring have a greater role in routine monitoring.

CONCLUSIONS

The findings of Study One and Two demonstrated that AE personnel believed that they had options to adequately control patients' pain during air transfer. However, a robust mechanism to provide auditable evidence of pain management in practice was lacking. Therefore, any potential claims by patients reporting to have experienced pain during AE could not be fully investigated at that time. Consequently, standard AE documentation required immediate review. Furthermore, a training package associated with promoting pain management as the "fifth vital sign" was required to ensure compliance with the revised documentation. This training was extended to deploying Aeromedical Evacuation Liaison Officers (AELO) and FNs to ensure compliance throughout the AE chain, which incorporates all operational theaters. A primary role of the AELO is to provide the interface between the originating medical facility in overseas locations and the AE Control Center in the UK.

These processes served as interim measures until the implementation of PGDs. Changes to the AE paperwork were to be re-evaluated after 6 months to establish if the documented management of pain had improved and to ensure educational programs had been effective.

STUDY THREE
Aim

The audit in Study Two was repeated to establish if the training program had delivered a change in behavior.

Method

All flight folders completed during May and June 2008 were included in the audit, which captured 283 patients on strategic flights from all destinations and created a manageable dataset for the auditor. Furthermore, 3 months had elapsed since the completion of the training program, which generated a credible interpretation of its efficacy by representing the standard of information retained over time.

Findings

The findings have been illustrated in **Table 3** in tabular format to permit ease of comparison to the data collated in June 2007. The data were further subdivided by operational theater to establish if particular training requirements were evident.

Discussion

The number of patient flight folders incorporated in this audit (283) was more than double that undertaken previously (140) to increase confidence in the findings. The decision to audit patients transferred during May and June 2008 was based on a period of time following the pain management training program to permit:

1. A locally produced pain assessment chart to be produced and implemented.
2. The opportunity for conveyed information standards to be distributed.

Comparing datasets that comprised different pain scoring systems was problematic; therefore, albeit an assumption, a pain score above 3 on the 0 to 10 scale was acknowledgment that the patients had experienced a mild level of pain, which would correlate with a score of 1 on the 0 to 3 scale. The percentage of patients with documented pain scores increased from 44% in June 2007 to 73% in July 2008; and the percentage of patients with no mention of pain management in their flight folders decreased from 42% to 14%, respectively. These figures would seem to reflect a significant increase in AE personnel's compliance with pain-assessment documentation standards. Marked improvement has also been achieved in the percentage of patients with their pain mentioned in the text of the notes but not as a score (from 14% to 8%), the percentage of battle-injured patients with documented pain assessment (from 54% to 92%), and non-battle injured patients (from 36% to 72%).

The number of patients in the June 2007 dataset sustaining battle injuries was 30% compared with 8% in the July 08 dataset, which is echoed by the percentage of

Table 3
Study three findings

Ser	Question	June 2007 Audit	July 2008 Audit	July 2008 Audit		
				UK-Based Strat	Deployed HERRICK	Deployed TELIC
1	Number of flight folders audited	140	283	149	86	48
2	Number of battle-injured patients	42	24	1	22	1
3	Percentage of total patients prescribed at least one form of analgesia	71%	56%	48%	69%	58%
4	Percentage of total patients with documented pain scores	44%	73%	81%	55%	81%
5	Percentage of patients with pain mentioned in the text but not scored	14%	8%	4%	16%	8%
6	Percentage of battle-injured patients with documented pain assessment	54%	92%	100%	91%	100%
7	Percentage of non-battle-injured patients with documented pain assessment	36%	72%	71%	47%	87%
8	Number of patients with pain documented as ≤ 3 (0–10 scale)	46 (33%)				
9	Number of patients with pain documented as ≤ 1 (0–3 scale)		173 (61%)	104 (70%)	40 (47%)	29 (60%)
10	Number of patients with pain documented as > 3 (0–10 scale)	15 (11%)				
11	Number of patients with pain documented as 2 or 3 (0–3 scale)		33 (12%)	16 (11%)	7 (8%)	10 (21%)
12	Percentage of patients with no mention of pain management in their flight folder	42%	14%	15%	16%	10%

patients in each audit that were prescribed one or more forms of analgesia (71% in 2007 and 56% in 2008) and a greater percentage (61%) experiencing none-to-mild pain in the most recent audit compared with 33% in 2007. Notwithstanding the reduction of patients presenting with the more obvious clinical indicators of pain in July 2008, the documentation is far more robust and suggests a greater awareness of the need to assess and reassess pain during flight. However, the standard demanded by the AE pain-management training program is that all AE patients must have their level of pain assessed, which includes psychiatric patients.

Scrutiny of the July 2008 data established that 8% of the Op HERRICK (Afghanistan) patients and 6% of the Op TELIC (Iraq) patients were psychiatric cases; however, none of these had any mention of pain assessment in their flight folders. The UK-based strategic dataset (excluding patients from Ops TELIC and HERRICK) in this small-scale study comprised 11% psychiatric patients and, of these, 38% had their pain assessments documented. This suggests that patients who do not present with physical pain are less likely to have this aspect of their care assessed during evacuation. However, the training program appears to have raised an awareness of pain scoring among AE Squadron personnel. It could also improve awareness for the management of psychiatric patients among those in deployed roles via the Psychiatric Aeromedical Evacuation Liaison Officer (PAELO).

The July 2008 audit permitted the discrimination of pain documentation standards in three specific strategic AE roles: UK-based, Op HERRICK, and Op TELIC. It was proposed that delivering training to the AE Squadron personnel for them to disseminate to operational environments via Standard Operating Procedures and the ground phase of AE training was the most expeditious and achievable platform to raise awareness and improve practice. This theory is corroborated by the findings, which illustrate personnel have significantly improved their practice.

Study Three suggests the greatest gap in compliance with AE patient pain-management documentation occurs in the deployed teams on Op HERRICK. The findings reflect that 55% of patients had documented pain scores and demonstrated only an 11% improvement in practice when compared with 44% in 07. The UK-based and Op TELIC teams demonstrated a 37% improvement in practice. Only 47% of Op HERRICK non-battle injured patients had documented pain assessment and, with only an 11% improvement, this was the lowest level of compliance when compared with UK-based and Op TELIC teams. In essence, this specific AE deployed asset has the most improvement to make and the study permits a more focused approach for remedial action.

SUMMARY

This audit has demonstrated a significant improvement in AE personnel's provision of robust pain assessment and documentation during patients' air transfer; this is an indication of the initial training program's effectiveness. However, further improvements are required to achieve the standard that all patients have a pain assessment conducted before flight and regularly thereafter if clinically indicated.

The Registered Mental Nurse cadre has responded well to the training program implemented on the AE Squadron and, owing to the level of noncompliance within this specialty, it would be beneficial for the PAELO to instruct personnel within their area of responsibility before their deployments. Similarly, this robust training could be delivered by the AELO to deployed Op HERRICK and Op TELIC teams to further improve documentation standards.

The regular turn-around of AE Squadron personnel warrants the training program being repeated every 6 months to ensure standards continue to improve. An additional audit is scheduled to take place in July 2009, which will continue the monitoring of changes in the robustness of practitioners' documentation behavior.

REFERENCES

1. Belanger HG, Scholten J, Curtiss G, et al. Utility of mechanism-of-injury-based assessment and treatment: blast injury program case illustration. J Rehabil Res Dev 2005;42(4):403–12.
2. Ficke JR, Pollak AN. Extremity war injuries: development of clinical treatment principles. J Am Acad Orthop Surg 2007;15:590–5.
3. Gould TH, Crosby DL, Harmer M, et al. Policy for controlling pain after surgery: effect of sequential changes in management. Br Med J 1992;305:1187–93.

Index

Note: Page numbers of article titles are in **boldface** type.

Nurs Clin N Am 45 (2010) 261–269
doi:10.1016/S0029-6465(10)00048-4
0029-6465/10/$ – see front matter © 2010 Elsevier Inc. All rights reserved.

nursing.theclinics.com

Moving?

Make sure your subscription moves with you!

To notify us of your new address, find your **Clinics Account Number** (located on your mailing label above your name), and contact customer service at:

Email: journalscustomerservice-usa@elsevier.com

800-654-2452 (subscribers in the U.S. & Canada)
314-447-8871 (subscribers outside of the U.S. & Canada)

Fax number: 314-447-8029

Elsevier Health Sciences Division
Subscription Customer Service
3251 Riverport Lane
Maryland Heights, MO 63043

*To ensure uninterrupted delivery of your subscription, please notify us at least 4 weeks in advance of move.